Brigid McConville is an award-winning health journalist and author of many books in this area.

Dr Rajendra Sharma is an acclaimed practitioner and author of *The Element Family Encyclopaedia of Health*.

YOUR CHILD SERIES

A series of books containing easy-to-follow, practical advice for the parents of children with a variety of illnesses or conditions.

Each book provides a clear overview of the situation, explaining essential information about the illness or condition and outlining the practical steps parents can take to help understand, support and care for their child, the rest of the family as well as themselves. Guiding parents through the conventional, the complementary and the alternative approaches which are available, these books cater for children of all ages, ranging from babies to teenagers, and enable the whole family to move forward in a positive way.

Titles in the Your Child series:

Your Child: Allergies by Brigid McConville with Dr Rajendra Sharma
Your Child: Asthma by Erika Harvey
Your Child: Bullying by Jenny Alexander
Your Child: Diabetes by Catherine Steven
Your Child: Dyslexia by Robin Temple
Your Child: Eczema by Maggie Jones
Your Child: Epilepsy by Fiona Marshall
Your Child: Headaches & Migraine by Maggie Jones

YOUR CHILD

Allergies

Practical and Easy-to-Follow Advice

Brigid McConville
with Dr Rajendra Sharma MB, BCh,
LRCP&S[I], MRCH, MFHom

ELEMENT
Shaftesbury, Dorset • Boston, Massachusetts
Melbourne, Victoria

© Element Books Limited 1999
Text © Brigid McConville 1999

First published in the UK in 1999 by
Element Books Limited
Shaftesbury, Dorset SP7 8BP

Published in the USA in 1999 by
Element Books, Inc.
160 North Washington Street
Boston, MA 02114

Published in Australia in 1999 by
Element Books and distributed
by Penguin Australia Limited
487 Maroondah Highway, Ringwood,
Victoria 3134

Cover photograph © Image Bank
Cover design by Slatter-Anderson
Design by Roger Lightfoot
Phototypeset by Intype London Ltd
Printed and bound in Great Britain by
Creative Print and Design (Wales), Ebbw Vale

British Library Cataloguing in Publication
data available

Library of Congress Cataloging in Publication
data available

ISBN 1 86204 499 6

Contents

Introduction   vii

1   What is Allergy?   1
2   Helping Your Child   13
3   The Emotional Aspects   25
4   Conventional Treatments   37
5   Complementary Therapies   53
6   As They Grow   79

Conclusion   93
Appendix   95
Further Reading   99
Useful Addresses   101
Index   109

Introduction

'It all started when Jason was one. After our Christmas party his whole face swelled up and his lips were very puffy. He was very upset and we found it alarming too, but I didn't know why it had happened. It was only later – after another more serious allergy attack – that I realized he had reacted to a dish of nuts which he had been handing around at the party.'

This is how Sally, Jason's mother, describes the first time that he experienced a serious allergic reaction. Her child's distress and her concern – particularly about not knowing what was happening to her son – are very common in families in which a child has an allergy or intolerance, especially a serious reaction like Jason's to nuts.

The next attack came when Jason was one and a half. He was at home with his mother at the time and Sally remembers that this one was even more alarming: 'Jason ate a chocolate from a selection box which had a brazil nut in the centre. Within minutes his voice had gone, he had been sick, there were weals all over his body and he had stomach cramps. I rang my husband, who is a doctor, but he was on call and I couldn't get hold of him. I then rang my brother who is a dentist, but I couldn't get hold of him either. I had no idea what the problem was; this happened 10 years ago and I had never heard of nut allergies. I waited, and fortunately, within about half an hour his symptoms had settled down.' But when Sally took Jason to their family doctor the next morning she realized that her son may have had a narrow escape: 'The doctor told me that Jason had had a severe allergic reaction and that I should have called an ambulance straight away. I still wake up in the night sometimes, thinking of what might have happened . . .'

Jason's doctor referred him to a specialist who discovered that he was in fact very allergic to walnuts, peanuts and – especially – brazil nuts. Sally has discovered since then that he also reacts to certain other substances: 'Jason is allergic to cats; whenever he comes into contact with them he becomes wheezy and breathless. Certain washing powders also cause him to react: he comes out in a rash all over.'

Sally doesn't know why her son has these allergic responses, but she is well aware that it is a common problem: 'Allergies and intolerances don't run in my family or in my husband's; we just don't know where it comes from, but there certainly seems to be a lot more of it about these days. Three of Jason's friends have allergies – including asthma – whereas it seemed quite rare when I was a child.'

We now know that babies can be sensitized to foods eaten by their mothers while still in the womb, and also by food molecules which find their way into the mother's breastmilk. Peanuts tend to cause the most dangerous reactions, whereas cow's milk is the most common culprit – and there are many other foods which can set up long-term problems too.

■ You are not alone

As both Sally and Jason know from experience, many children today – Jason's friends amongst them – suffer from allergies and intolerances. Not all instances are as dramatic and life-threatening as his, but whether they show up as eczema, asthma, hayfever, hives or another kind of reaction, they can have a big impact on day-to-day life.

The rate at which children suffer allergies and intolerances has risen markedly over the last 30 years too. Asthma alone now affects at least one in seven children in the UK. Australia tops the league with an extraordinary one in three children having symptoms of asthma.

According to the UK charity Action Against Allergy, there has also been a big increase in cases of allergy and intolerances in babies and small children. AAA cites a Finnish study which reported that 19 per cent of babies were found to be allergic at 12 months, 27 per cent at 3 years and 8 per cent at 6 years. And as allergy often goes unrecognized by doctors, the true numbers are likely to be much higher.

But what are the reasons for this dramatic rise? There is no simple or single answer, but allergies and intolerances seem to be very much a man-made disease. They are common in the developed Western world, but rare in countries without our technologies, industries, pollution, processed food – and medicines. Complementary practitioners point out that the increase has coincided with the rise in the use of antibiotics.

Another reason for the upsurge could be that we are constantly surrounded by substances – in our food, in the air we breathe, in our homes – which cause reactions in our bodies. It's possible that over hundreds of thousands of years, the human body had developed the ability to defend itself against natural compounds – but that we have fewer defences against the many new and artificial substances that we have created in the modern world.

In addition, our diet has changed dramatically since the Second World War and we now eat an immense range of foods – imported and processed – which either didn't exist or were completely unobtainable earlier this century. No one yet knows what modern food production is really doing to our health. And the issue of genetically modified foodstuffs only adds to our concern.

Stress also makes us more susceptible to allergies and

intolerances, and while we may not be experiencing more stress than our ancestors (who often lived very hard lives indeed), our modern sedentary way of life means that stress tends to build up inside us. Instead of running or fighting when stressed as nature intended, we are more often stuck behind a desk or the wheel of a car.

But the good news is that allergies or intolerances do not have to dominate your life, or the life of your family. Many children grow out of them in the course of time and it is possible – once you have identified them (as Jason and Sally did) – to avoid many of the substances and foods which cause them.

With some sorts of allergy – such as asthma – modern medicine offers drugs to control some of the symptoms (inhalers, for instance). These can be lifesaving – and you should never underestimate the dangers of a serious allergy – but they don't address the causes of the allergy or intolerance.

Complementary therapies take a different approach, not only eliminating the triggers of allergies and intolerances but looking for the reasons behind them and addressing the roots of the problem. A wide range of therapies (detailed later in this book) can help regulate your child's immune system – making her less susceptible to a whole range of illnesses, including allergies and intolerances. In some cases, a prescribed course of complementary therapy can put an end to them once and for all.

This book is about how *you* can make a difference to your child's allergies or intolerances. It not only provides you with the information you need about the symptoms and causes, but also suggests many practical ways to tackle them and to feel more in control of the situation. As a parent you have a vital role to play in identifying the foods and other substances which trigger allergies or intolerances in your child. You are also better placed than anyone else to make the necessary changes in your child's diet and environment which are needed to prevent them.

The following chapters provide you with clear information about the conventional medical treatments for allergies and intolerances, and also include a comprehensive guide to the wide range of complementary therapies now available – with suggestions about which of these are most likely to help your child. The book looks at allergies and intolerances not simply as a set of symptoms, but as a wider problem which has an effect on – and is rooted in – our day-to-day lives.

For, as the many parents interviewed in this book have testified, coping with allergies or intolerances can be a stressful business not only for your child, but for you and your whole family. From the time that she is a baby, they can make life that much more complicated and worrying. As babies grow into toddlers and then schoolchildren, venturing more and more into the outside world, allergies and intolerances can also have an impact on school, social and family life. But you can deal with the problems of allergies and intolerances in a positive way, keeping an open mind about treatments both orthodox and complementary, looking after yourself as well as your child, and above all, staying relaxed, well informed and on top of things!

Note: 'He' and 'she' have been used to describe your child in alternate chapters to avoid the more cumbersome 'he or she'.

—

Chapter One

What is Allergy?

Your children are sitting around the kitchen table with a couple of their friends, ready for their evening meal. You serve up the pizza, the pasta, or fish dish. Then one of your young visitors pipes up: 'I can't eat that; I'm allergic to tomatoes/ cheese/ fish' – or whatever it might be. For a moment you are stumped. 'Allergy' is a word that crops up so often these days and in such different circumstances. On the one hand we know that it can be very serious, even fatal. Some children – like Jason in the Introduction – have allergies to nuts which are so severe that even the slightest contact is potentially fatal (this is called an anaphylactic reaction, see also p.49). On the other hand there are children who claim 'I'm allergic to that' because they just don't like what has appeared on the table! But clearly, the last thing you want to do is to encourage a child to eat something which is going to make them ill.

So what exactly is allergy? Technically speaking, allergy is an overreaction by the body's defences (immune system) to a foreign body (antigen) which causes a range of symptoms anywhere in the body. These may be immediate, or delayed for up to 72 hours. If this sounds a bit vague, that's because allergy takes many forms, has a wide variety of symptoms – and doctors still don't entirely agree as to what it's all about. Complementary practitioners, too, have many theories – some widely accepted, others still controversial – as to what allergies are and how you can tackle them.

Common forms of allergy often suffered by children include asthma, eczema, hayfever and hives (urticaria). All of these are reactions to substances that we eat, drink, touch, or breathe in.

Allergic reactions are rather like your body's response to any foreign substance – be they germs or splinters. Normally, your body responds with a range of defences, called antibodies, to fight off any invader. Familiar signs of this fight in your body include swelling, redness and fever – all healthy indications that your immune system is at work. If you are prone to allergies however, your immune system overdoes it, fighting off 'invaders' (such as nuts or pollen) which otherwise wouldn't do you any harm. And once your body has mistaken these harmless substances for 'the enemy' it 'remembers' what happened the last time and sets up a system for making the antibodies quickly – in case the 'invader' returns.

The most common of these antibodies is called immunoglobulin E (IgE) and it becomes active chiefly in the blood, the mucous membranes of the nose, throat and mouth, and in the skin. When the 'enemy' shows up again, IgE sets off a release of chemicals in the body. The best known of these chemicals is called histamine, and it (together with other chemicals) causes those immediate symptoms of allergy with which we are all familiar – including rashes, itching, sneezing, wheezing, runny nose and eyes, bronchial spasm, hives, vomiting and tingling of the mouth. Histamine is made by the body whenever it is injured or under attack from infection. It increases the size of the blood vessels so that blood can quickly get to damaged tissue in order to begin repair.

■ WHAT IS AN INTOLERANCE?

At this point it is worth noting the difference between an 'allergy' and an 'intolerance' or 'sensitivity'. The dividing line is in fact rather blurred, so much so that 'intolerance' is sometimes called 'psuedo-allergy'.

Intolerance, like allergy, happens when the body's immune system overreacts, but the process is slower and the symptoms not so obvious. With allergy the response is often quick and noticeable immediately or at least within hours, and always within 72 hours. If your child is allergic to cats for instance, you will probably be able to tell that there is a cat in the room (or even that a cat has been in the room) because your child's eyes and nose will start to run within minutes. In contrast, an intolerance can take months, even years, to develop.

But intolerance is not only slower, it is also more difficult to diagnose. Allergies can usually be detected by a simple skin or blood test. Intolerances, by contrast, are hard to link up to a cause, and doctors regard them with much more scepticism.

The mechanism of an intolerance may be different from that of allergy too. In allergy, the body's defences fight an 'invader'. With intolerance, it may be an ingredient in food which directly harms or irritates the body, such as gluten in cereals, proteins in cheese or fish, or caffeine in coffee, tea, cola drinks and chocolate. Intolerances do not necessarily produce a histamine reaction.

Intolerance may also show up in different ways: for example, children who are sensitive to food additives may become hyperactive. Symptoms in all age groups may include changes in concentration, memory, thinking and behaviour, causing mood swings and/or anxiety. Or symptoms of intolerance may show up as chronic illnesses, such as irritable bowel syndrome or chronic fatigue syndrome.

One of the more controversial symptoms of food sensitivity

is hyperactivity, sometimes known as Hyperkinetic Syndrome (also Attention Deficit Disorder or Attention Deficit and Hyperkinetic Disorder) which is thought to affect from 1 to 20 per cent of children. Boys for some reason are five times more prone to it (see also Chapter 6).

The latest research shows that many hyperactive children are sensitive not only to the commonly eaten foods and food additives but also to a range of allergens, including pollen, dust and chemicals. It could be that the dramatic increase in hyperactivity in recent years is linked to the rise in our consumption of additive-packed convenience and fast foods.

Unfortunately, conventional doctors are often highly sceptical when it comes to food sensitivities and food allergy (other than extreme reactions like anaphylaxsis). Many mothers of colicky babies will know how frustrating it is to be told their baby will 'soon grow out of it' – or worse, that their baby is simply reacting to their own nervous inadequacy in the parenting department! With older children, too, parents may have difficulty in being taken seriously when they suspect their child is reacting badly to certain foods.

In the past decade however, more and more doctors have become alert to the real possibility that many common ailments affecting babies and small children can be caused by sensitivity to foods as many complementary practitioners already acknowledge. From colic and eczema to glue ear and headaches, from asthma and persistent runny noses to behavioural problems and tummy aches – all may be caused by certain foods or additives in foods.

Common symptoms of intolerance
- Tiredness
- Aching muscles
- Migraine
- Mouth ulcers
- Water retention

- Nausea and vomiting
- Gastric and duodenal ulcers
- Wind and bloating
- Irritable bowel syndrome
- Constipation
- Rheumatoid arthritis
- Anxiety
- Depression
- Hyperactivity in children
- Attention deficit disorder

Some children are intolerant to certain foods because they lack the physical ability to cope with them. For instance, many people react badly to dairy products because they can't digest them properly. This is because many of us have a shortage of the enzyme lactase. Other sensitivities or intolerances may be triggered by an overexposure to pollutants, such as chemicals or detergents. This could be because the body is so busy fighting chemicals that the immune system is compromised and it ignores other 'invaders'. Alternatively, it could be because the body's defences becomes overactive and start to attack molecules which it shouldn't.

Another possible cause of food intolerance is Leaky Gut Syndrome. Your small intestine is a kind of sieve which should allow only the breakdown products of digestion into your blood-stream (for instance amino acids and peptides – broken down from proteins). Larger particles of protein, carbohydrate and fat are usually 'sieved out' so that they don't get into the blood. This is because your body may react to these as 'the enemy' with an attack response from your immune system. However, in Leaky Gut Syndrome, this sieve mechanism breaks down so that foods that have not been digested fully are absorbed into the bloodstream. This syndrome may have a number of causes, ranging from foods which inflame the bowels, to yeasts, viruses, bacteria, antibiotics – or even stress.

One theory is that certain drugs, including headache tablets, as well as an over-growth of the yeast organism *Candida albicans*, can cause this leaky effect by making 'holes' in the walls of the gut. Leaky Gut Syndrome may, therefore, be at the root of many food allergies.

CAUSES OF ALLERGY

The whole subject of allergy and intolerance is a controversial one – especially when it comes to identifying causes. Partly this is because we simply don't know all the answers to how and why allergies and intolerances occur and partly because different practitioners can take very different approaches in treatment. Yet we can be sure of some things: certainly, allergy and/or intolerance can run in the family; it can also be caused by sensitivity to certain foods; it can be caused by a sensitivity to common allergens, such as pollen, dust mite faeces and chemicals; and it can also be brought on and exacerbated by extreme stress.

Is pollution to blame?

In recent years there has been a significant increase in the amount of allergies and intolerances that we suffer, especially in the Western, industrialized world. Estimates vary but some say that up to a quarter of people in the West suffer from allergies and/or intolerances at some time in their lives. In less developed countries, however, allergies like asthma and hayfever are much rarer.

Why should this be? Again, there is no definitive proof, but the emerging concensus is that environmental pollution is an important factor. When it comes to common allergies like asthma, pollution is known to be a significant trigger for the allergic response.

Not only the air that we breathe, but also our water and our food is often contaminated by a certain level of chemicals, such as pesticides, additives and artificial colourings. On a daily basis we come into contact with toxins too: heavy metals in petrol fumes, mercury in tooth fillings, chemicals in cosmetics and detergents. Our bodies are constantly having to defend themselves against harmful substances to such an extent that they sometimes become overloaded.

Diet: what you eat, you are

Our modern diet is highly refined, often consisting of foods which have been stored and processed, often leaving us deficient in the many essential vitamins and minerals that our bodies need to stay healthy. A low level of vital nutrients can lead to a weakened immune system which, in turn, is linked to allergy. The chances are that if your child eats a lot of refined foods, he will be more prone to developing an allergy.

Another important cause of allergies is the decline of breast-feeding in the Western world. Breast really is best, because:

- Breastfeeding primes your baby's gut and immune system (which remain immature until one year), making it less likely that he will develop an allergy.
- Nutritionally, this is the best possible food for your baby, matching his every and ever-changing need(s).
- Formula milk and giving solids in the first year of life can cause allergies in sensitive children.

Most infant formulas are based on cow's milk which can cause an allergic reaction. In one scientific study of 1,700 babies in maternity wards, (quoted by Professor Jonathon Brostoff in his book *The Complete Guide to Food Allergy and Intolerance*) 1,500 were given 'supplementary' feeds in hospital, while 200 were not. Of this group of babies, 39 developed an allergy to cow's milk; there were no allergies to cow's milk in the group of 200 which were exclusively breastfed.

Some babies – especially those with cow's milk allergies in their families – are given formula milk derived from soya. This can be prescribed by your doctor, and may effectively clear up symptoms of allergy to cow's milk, but soya itself can cause an allergic reaction, espcially if the mother has eaten soya products (and soya flour is in many foods) during pregnancy.

There are various reasons for this kind of reaction in babies. Not only do babies have highly 'absorbent' bowels, but they also don't produce as much pancreatic enzyme as older children or adults; their bowel bacteria are also relatively undeveloped. All this means that a baby's bowel will therefore be absorbing large, undigested molecules, which the body then mistakes for an 'invader' – triggering an allergic response.

The holistic view

Another theory is that allergies and intolerances are a sign that the body's immune system is overworked. Some complementary practitioners argue that allergy and/or intolerance occurs when the body is already in battle mode, primed to fight a condition somewhere else – that you may or may not know about. For instance, if your child shows symptoms of hayfever in the summer, it could be that he has an underlying food allergy or intolerance, without which he wouldn't react to pollen.

This 'holistic' theory could explain why some of us react allergically and some of us do not – even though we all come into contact with much the same foods and substances. Even within families with similarly inherited traits, some children will be allergic or intolerant and others not.

There is also strong evidence to suggest that allergies and intolerances are linked to what goes on in our psyche. We are all increasingly aware these days that the workings of the mind/

spirit/ emotions have a very powerful influence on our bodies. This influence is so great that in some people hayfever can be triggered by flowers which are in fact artificial.

Too much stress also puts a strain on our bodies and makes us more susceptible to suffering the symptoms not only of allergy, but also of food intolerance.

Do allergies run in the family?

Heredity seems to play a part in who gets allergies and/or intolerances. If you or your child's other parent suffers from allergies, then your children have a higher than usual chance (around 30 per cent) of suffering from them too. If you and your child's other parent are both allergic, this risk goes up to around 60 per cent.

This inherited predispostion or tendency to be allergic is called 'atopy' – hence the terms 'atopic asthma', 'atopic eczema', and so on. Allergy may show up in your family in different forms too; you might have asthma, while one child has eczema and another has hayfever.

This family tendency to suffer from allergies and/or intolerances may be more than a matter of straightforward genetics however. Recent studies which have looked at siblings and their childhood illnesses suggest that the more we are exposed to infections, the less likely we are to develop allergies. Children who have older brothers and sisters – and who are introduced that way to more childhood infections – tend to suffer less from allergy than the first born.

Your child's risk of developing an allergy or intolerance
- If either you or your partner has an allergy and/or intolerance, your child has a 20–30 per cent chance of being predisposed to allergy.
- If both you and your partner are allergic and/or intolerant, your child has a 40–60 per cent chance of being predisposed to allergy.

- If you and your partner both have the same allergy and/or
  intolerance, your child has a 70 per cent chance of
  developing that allergy.

  But note: a third of children with allergies are born into families
  in which neither parent has noticed any allergic symptoms in
  themselves. From *The Complete Guide to Food Allergy and
  Intolerance* by Professor Jonathan Brostoff

It seems likely that if your child's body learns to fight infections
when he is young, it is less likely to go overboard with an
allergic response later on. This is the reasoning behind the view
that the rise in allergies amongst children may be linked to
vaccinations.

It could be that vaccinations – by preventing many common
childhood illnesses – stop your child's body from getting his
immune system into full swing. Some complementary practitioners argue that we should reconsider our mass vaccination
programme against measles, mumps and rubella, for example,
on the basis that the damage – and sometimes death – caused
by asthma outweighs the advantages of vaccinations.

Case Study

Tim, aged five, suffers from allergies including eczema. His
mother believes that they began after a course of routine
vaccinations:

'I worry that it was the injections he had as a baby which
started it off – either that or perhaps the suspension they use
in the injections. He was fine until he was three months old
and then he had the usual jabs. As soon as that happened his
cradle cap turned into dermatitis of the head, all yellow and
flakey but red underneath. Within two weeks of the jabs it
had spread all over his body, covering him completely.

Sometimes his skin splits and then it is very sore. It goes
in a cycle; first it gets red and hot. Then white spots develop
which is a sign of infection. Then he gets red raw patches
and becomes feverish. At that point he needs antibiotics.

At first, our doctor prescribed cortisone cream, but we were reluctant to use it because of the potential side-effects on a small baby. We took him to a homeopathic hospital where he was given the remedy silica. It didn't do anything remarkable, but we felt that we were doing *something*.

Since then we've made sure he has a very healthy, whole-food diet. We do eat fish but he has never eaten meat and we avoid all dairy products.

Simply taking control of the situation by giving him a good diet and finding out all we can has helped. We use a lot of emollients in the bath and we found that evening primrose oil cream was a help. When he is in the bath I put a handful of porridge oats in a sock into the water; that works really well and I can also clean him with it.

I also worry that stress is part of it. Perhaps if I had not been working at the time I would have done some research and would have avoided giving him the vaccinations. I feel frustrated now that I didn't do that.

But I do believe you cannot let the allergy dictate how you live your life. You have to hold out, try to keep him well and hope that it will pass. I don't let the eczema stop him from doing anything. I let him play in the sand and then doctor him when he comes home. He doesn't want it to stop him from doing things, so I let him carry on and sort out any problems later. I do believe he will grow out of it in time.'

Whatever the cause of your child's allergy or intolerance, however, the trick is to discover what triggers it off so that you can take avoiding action and stay in control of the situation. In the next chapter, we hear from other parents who have been following the clues down the allergy trail.

Chapter Two

Helping Your Child

For most parents, the process of asking whether or not their children are allergic and/or intolerant begins when the children are very young, often when they are still babies. For first-time parents, especially, this can be a time of great stress as they struggle to find out exactly what is going on.

Ann looks back on the early months of her son George's life as a kind of waking nightmare for them both – because he not only cried constantly but never slept for more than two hours at a stretch: 'It started when George was a few months old. He had colic, which meant lots of screaming and not sleeping properly. Half an hour after a feed he would start to scream. I had to walk the floor with him for an hour or more, my hand pressing on his tummy; I couldn't put him down. I was so tired and so desperate that I nearly threw him down the stairs one night. I also became a hermit: I couldn't go out anywhere without him because I couldn't leave him with anyone. I was too exhausted to eat properly myself and I was very afraid that my breastmilk might dry up, so I drank a lot of cow's milk in the belief that it would be good for me and for breastfeeding George.'

Only later did Ann discover that the cow's milk might be making George's colic even worse. She decided to take George to the doctor but he told her not to worry, it was 'just infant colic'. 'He made me feel as if I was making a great fuss about nothing. But the colic and screaming and sleeplessness just went on and on. But in a way you get used to it and I thought that was just the way he was.'

Then when George was about six-months-old Ann noticed a pattern: 'He was on solid food by then and I realized that on some days he was better than on others. One thing that made it a lot worse was mashed potatoes with cheese. After that he wouldn't sleep, was always on the move and had to be picked up by me constantly. He was a wreck and so was I.'

Ann started to wonder if food might be at the root of her child's problems and so she read up on the subject. 'From what I could find in books, it seemed to me that the culprit could be cow's milk, so I followed what he ate and how he reacted day by day.' When Ann felt fairly sure about her theory, she went back to her doctor and told him about her suspicions. 'He just said "I doubt it". So I spoke to the nurse in the child clinic who also dismissed the whole idea.'

But Ann is an independent-minded person and so she shrugged off this dismissal and decided to put her ideas to the test. 'I took George off cow's milk for a week and gave him goat's milk instead. Unfortunately, it wasn't long enough to make any difference – but I didn't know that at the time.'

Then one day when George was nearly one, Ann gave him some chocolate buttons for the first time, as a treat. Within an hour he was in extreme distress. 'His stools turned black. I called the doctor and I asked my mother to get hold of some goat's milk for him. She came in the back door at exactly the same moment as the doctor came in the front. He took one look at George and said "take him to hospital".'

By the time George was examined in hospital he had lost over half of his red blood cells through internal bleeding – hence the black colour of his nappies.

'I kept saying to the doctors and nurses "I think he's allergic to cow's milk",' says Ann, 'but they still gave him a glass of milk a day. We sat there for two days in the hospital, trying to keep a drip in his arm. It was just awful. The hospital thought it might be an ulcer and they wanted to try a whole battery of tests.'

But having already endured attempts to get a syringe into her baby's arm, Ann refused to allow any more intrusive procedures, signed a form and took George home. She still feels annoyed and hurt that the hospital staff accused her of wanting to take her son home simply because it was his birthday. 'When we got home I burst into tears. I was heavily pregnant with my second child and terrified that George was just going to drop dead.'

But he didn't. On the contrary. Ann took him off all cow's milk products, and gradually, he stopped screaming, started sleeping – and turned into a different child. George is now a happy, healthy, boy though he still reacts badly when he eats certain foods or has fizzy drinks.

ALLERGY AND INTOLERANCE: IDENTIFYING THE CULPRITS

Ann's story has a positive ending, but unfortunately, she – like many other parents of allergic children – had to go through many months of worry before she found the cause of her child's health problems. Ann found her own solution by carefully observing her child and noting what made him better or worse, over a period of time. By identifying and then eliminating the main suspect – cow's milk, in this case – from George's diet, she brought about a dramatic improvement in his health and well-being – not to mention her own peace of mind and stress levels.

Like Ann, there is a great deal you can do, too, in terms of self-help to identify, prevent and alleviate the symptoms. The first step is to identify the factor – or factors – which trigger your child's allergy and/or intolerance.

It can help to keep a diary of everything your child eats and drinks from day to day as well as other ordinary details of her life. Note when the symptoms come on and anything that makes them better or worse. This will help you spot the links between her allergic and/or intolerance reaction and its cause. For instance, has she been playing at a friend's house where a cat lives? Has she had fizzy drinks or sweets at a party? These can all be clues to which substance triggers your child's allergy.

Similarly, are there any smells which your child can't abide, or any foods that she really likes to eat – over and over again? Paradoxically, we often crave foods to which we are intolerant. Homeopaths believe that this is because the body reacts to make itself better whenever possible.

For instance, a cold virus causes the nose to produce mucus to trap the 'invader' – which we then remove when we blow our noses. Working on the same principle it could be that the body – recognizing a problem with a certain type of food – creates a craving for that food. By eating the food, we cause a reaction to occur, and the more we react, the more we are likely to recognize that this type of food is not good for us.

If the clues to your child's allergy add up to a signficiant pattern, you may be able to identify a suspect. If so, you have already won at least half the battle.

If you seriously think a certain type of food is causing your child's allergy or intolerance, you could start with one of these simple 'exclusion' diets:

■ The 'favourite foods' exclusion diet

1 Take your child's five favourite foods, *plus* the five foods which she eats most (these are likely to overlap), and cut them out of her diet for *at least six weeks.*

2 If you see no improvement, these foods are unlikely to be the source of the problem. If you *do* see an improvement, keep the diet up for *three months*.
3 At this point you could re-introduce these foods gradually. By now you child's body is likely to have 'forgotten' that one or more of these foods is 'the enemy', so she may be able to eat them again without her body rushing to the attack (an allergic response).
4 If she does respond allergically to re-introduced food, however, keep her off it for another *six weeks* and then try again. If again, she responds allergically, keep her off the food for a longer period of *around three months*. Alternatively, you may want to try complementary therapies, as described in Chapter five.

▓ The 'food group' exclusion diet

1 Pick a food group and cut out *all* varieties of food belonging to this group from your child's diet. For example: if the group is *grain*, eliminate wheat, rice, rye, corn, millet etc. If the group is *dairy*, eliminate every kind of food which comes from cows, such as milk, cheese, butter, yogurt, ice cream. Other food groups are listed below.
2 Keep up this diet for a 'test period' of *six weeks*. If you see no improvement, you are on the wrong trail. If you do see an improvement, carry on for *three months*, as above.
Note (If you are excluding animal protein from your child's diet, you should add in lentils, beans, soya and tofu in order to maintain good nutrition.)

With either of these exclusion diets your child may have 'withdrawal symptoms' from the foods she is no longer eating. These may include increased headaches and rashes, while pre-existing symptoms, such as tiredness and lethargy, may become worse.

These symptoms should only last for a few days however and are a sign that you are on the right track. You can help to reduce them by making sure that your child drinks plenty of plain water to flush out her system.

> **Simple guide to food groups**
> - **Dairy** Anything from a cow
> - **Grain** Wheat, rye, corn, millet, rice, barley
> - **Animal protein** Meat, fish, chicken, eggs, cheese
> - **Vegetable protein** Wholegrain cereals (including wholemeal bread), lentils, beans, tofu and soya
> - **Citrus** Oranges, lemons, grapefruit, limes
>
> (See Appendix for more details of food groups)
>
> You may want to try a more comprehensive test such as an Elimination Diet. When doing this with children, it is important to consult a qualified practitioner. Details of this diet are on p.40.

If you have a tough time explaining to your child why she has to give up so many of the foods she likes best, try telling her that – if the diet works – she may be able to enjoy them again soon without any nasty reactions!

These simple exclusion diets are suitable for children because while one food group or set of foods is excluded, there are plenty of alternatives to choose from. If you suspect your child is allergic or intolerant to food from different food groups, however, and you decide to try a more complicated exclusion diet, do consult a trained nutritionist first. A varied, well-balanced diet is particularly important for healthy growth in childhood.

> **Tackling Leaky Gut Syndrome**
> As we have seen, allergy begins when your child's body overreacts to a substance or allergen which it (wrongly) identifies as 'the enemy'. Most of these allergens (apart from those which are inhaled or absorbed through the skin) have been absorbed into the bloodstream through the bowel which has become 'leaky', usually after an inflammation. This means

that it fails to 'sieve out' larger food molecules which then get into the blood and set up the allergic reaction.

If your child has developed an allergy within two to three months of having a tummy upset, it is likely that her bowel has become 'leaky' and needs to be 'resealed' before she can overcome the allergic response. (If her bowel remains leaky, you could take her off dairy products for instance, only to find that she develops an allergy to something else, such as wheat.)

To reseal the gut, complementary practitioners may advise a course of high-dose acidophilus, according to the age of your child. If your child is under two, she may be given probifidus; after two, children may be given acidophilus, probifidus and other varieties of bifidus treatments.

It could also be that your child's body is not breaking down his food properly because she is short of the necessary pancreatic enzymes and/or hydrochloric acid in her gut. A complementary practitioner may suggest treatment to remedy these deficiencies.

Meanwhile it is important for your child to avoid foods which may inflame her bowel. These include highly refined sugars (which stimulate the wrong kind of bacterial growth in the gut), caffeine (found in colas, chocolate and chocolate drinks as well as tea and coffee), and spicy food (unless your child is already used to spices). It is also important to avoid antibiotics – which means not just prescribed medicines, but also all meat which is not from an organic source.

Antibiotics kill off our most prominent (healthy) bowel bacteria known as *Bifido lactobacillus*, leaving the more aggressive *E. coli* and streptococci that also colonize the bowel with more food to consume. They then multiply much more quickly and damage the bowel lining, potentially leading to Leaky Gut Syndrome.

This loss of bacteria can also encourage the growth of *Candida albicans* which can damage the bowel wall, as well as releasing chemicals which can make us feel unwell, while also promoting allergic responses.

▮ AVOIDING THE CULPRITS

▮ Home sweet home?

We have seen how you can identify – and avoid – certain allergens in the food your child eats, but how can you avoid those allergens which are part of our everyday environment?

The best place to start is in your home. Ironically, the harder you try to make your home into a warm and cosy haven for your children, the more likely you are to be contributing to their allergies and/or intolerances. For our modern, centrally heated, freshly painted, insulated and double-glazed homes – with their carefully tended gardens and beloved cat or dog – are the ideal breeding ground for a number of potent allergens. One of these is the house dust mite, a common trigger for allergies.

Dust mites are too small to spot without a microscope, and they live by eating the little bits of human skin that we all shed at the rate of one teaspoonful a day. It is their dung (which we breathe in when dust is disturbed) which can cause an allergic reaction.

No matter how houseproud you are, dust mites will make themselves at home in your carpets, curtains, sofas, beds, cushion and pillows, munching on the dust which inevitably gathers there. And the conditions which dust mites like the best for growing and breeding – namely warmth (around 25°C) and humidity (around 80 per cent) – are perfectly provided by central heating. Dust mites are particularly fond of bedding – which is kept warm and moist by your child's body all night long – and up to two million of them are likely to be living in your child's mattress alone!

But how can you make your home uncomfortable for the dust mite without making it too uncomfortable for your own family? It's easy enough to turn down the central heating and throw open the windows from time to time, but few of us would want to go without carpets, curtains and soft furnishings altogether, or to give up sleeping on a mattress!

Fortunately, there are ways to cut down on dust mite numbers without cutting out your home comforts entirely. Concentrating on your child's bedroom and your living room, try a combination of the following measures:

Cutting down on dust mite
1 Get rid of as many dust and dust mite havens (that is, carpets, curtains, sofas) as you can. Bare wood floorboards or vinyl can be very attractive and easy to keep clean. Plastic blow-up furniture is also very 'cool' with children these days, while blinds can be a stylish (and easy to wipe) alternative to curtains. If you must have carpets, choose short pile.
2 Cover your child's mattress, pillows and duvet or quilt (filled with man-made fibres, not feathers or down) with special barrier covers which you can buy from leading chemists/pharmacies or by mail order. If these are too expensive for you, simply double up on sheets and pillowcases on the basis that two are better than one at keeping mite particles at bay.
3 Wash any bedding that you can – such as blankets and duvets/quilts – at temperatures above 55°C every month to kill dust mites. Put your child's teddies or soft toys in the wash too or, if they aren't washable, put them in your freezer once a week to kill off mites.
4 Vacuum your floors – and soft furnishings if you can – once a day or as often as possible. Do use a good vacuum cleaner with air filters to prevent re-emission of particles (some vacuum cleaners simply puff dust straight back into the air of your home).
   A good vacuum cleaner will also have attachments for dusting – far better than stirring dust up with an old-fashioned 'duster' cloth or feather duster. Alternatively, try 'damp dusting' with a damp cloth and/or mop.
5 Mites love humidity, so keep your home cool and dry by opening windows or using an extractor fan when you are having a shower or cooking. (If your child is allergic to pollen, only open windows at night.) Weather permitting, dry your laundry outdoors rather than in drying machines or on radiators in your home.

▥ Animal allergens

Apart from the dust mite, there are other larger, more cuddly creatures which can also cause major problems at home for children with allergies. Cats, dogs, guinea pigs, hamsters, budgies – any furry or feathered creature in fact – can be a serious source of allergens in your home.

Your child may feel totally stricken at the thought of parting with her beloved pet, but doctors strongly recommend it! It may harden your heart to know that 40 per cent of children with asthma are sensitized to cat allergens, and once they are sensitized, even brief exposure to a cat can lead to a severe asthma attack. Cat allergen comes from cats' sweat glands and it can linger in rooms where a cat has been years after the animal has gone – which explains why your child may react even when the cat is no longer in the room.

Dogs are less of a problem when it comes to triggering allergies, with 10 to 15 per cent of children being sensitized to the dog's allergen. In dogs, the allergen is found in dander (dandruff), fur and saliva, and unfortunately, it doesn't matter whether dogs (or cats) are long- or short-haired: they are equally capable of causing allergies.

If you can't bear to give your pet away, try to keep it out of doors or confine it to the kitchen. If you do find an alternative home for it, clean thoroughly, preferably with a steam cleaner, wherever the animal might have been.

▥ HOME IMPROVEMENT DANGERS

The more you love your home and family, the more likely you are to put a lot of effort into making it as attractive as possible. Unfortunately, many of the processes and products we use in DIY and home improvements can also set off allergies.

Solvent-based paints, varnishes, cleaning fluids and sprays, glues and chemical treatments – all have the potential to cause a reaction in your child's sensitive skin or airways. You can, however, buy solvent-free emulsion paints and other DIY products from specialist suppliers (see Useful Addresses). As for cleaning, most environmentally friendly products (from your local health store or market), and even old-fashioned soap or soda crystals and water, will do a good job without the reactions caused by more commercial products.

Alternatively, it's worth asking yourself 'Does this job really have to be done?' Even if the answer is 'Yes', ask 'Does it have to be done now?' Many parents start 'nest building' with each new baby, yet avoiding allergens in pregnancy could be crucial to your child's future health.

There is one important exception: if your house has a damp problem, fix it as soon as possible. Damp breeds mould and mould spores are allergens. So do tackle that leaky roof or rising damp patch or dripping pipe. On the same basis, try to make sure your bathroom and kitchen are well ventilated and that your home is warm enough in the winter to prevent moisture from condensing on the walls.

IN YOUR GARDEN

What with dust mites and paint fumes and mould spores, you might want to take refuge in your garden as the safest place for an allergic child. But many gardens have grassy lawns, hedges, borders of trees – all the better to ambush your family not only with pollen but with yet more mould spores!

All is not lost, however. The concept of the Low Allergen Garden has been gaining ground for some years now. The idea is to organize your garden to cause the minimum of allergic reaction. Grasses, hedges, trees, mould-producing mulches and heavily scented pollinated flowers (like those of the daisy family) are out. Paved and/or gravelled areas with pot plants, trellises (to support climbing plants) and ground-cover plants (to cut down on pollen producing weeds) are in.

In the garden, timing is important too. If your child is allergic to pollen, encourage her to play there on dull, damp days and/or early mornings when the pollen count is low. If she is allergic to mould spores, avoid the damp days (when mould spores are released) and send her outside when the sun shines!

Chapter Three

The Emotional Aspects

Every parent of a child with an allergy and/or intolerance knows what a struggle it can be – not only to get to the root of the problem, but also to find the right kind of treatment. And, in the meantime, the whole family is affected by the day-to-day realities of living with the condition.

Always to the fore is concern, even fear, for your child. Will he be all right – not just today, but in the future, too? What if he has a severe reaction, like an asthma attack or even anaphylatic shock (see p.49) and you are not around to help him? What does it feel like to know that your child will be singled out from other children, made to feel that something is 'wrong' with him, excluded from certain meals and activities?

For allergy is not just a problem which affects your child's eyes or nose, lungs or bowels, but the mind and emotions, and so his feelings – and yours – too. Good health involves not just the body, but the whole person.

YOUR CHILD'S FEELINGS

Ask most children how they feel about having an allergy and/ or intolerance and the chances are they will be very matter of fact about it. After all, they say, allergies/intolerances are very common these days. So many of their friends have asthma now that having an inhaler is almost 'normal'. But children are by nature very adaptable and the fact that on the surface they seem to accept something without any fuss, doesn't mean that they aren't feeling it deeply.

Above all, children hate to feel different from their peers. To most adults, embarrassment is a passing emotion which we can usually joke about soon after; to sensitive children it can mean long-lasting and utter mortification. Anything that makes them look different – such as eczema on their hands or faces – or which excludes them from shared activities, can be a source of great stress. And stress, by undermining the immune system, can make allergies worse.

Another major issue for children is food. Most children love food in a way that adults have almost forgotten. Food is comfort and pleasure, sustenance and reward, fun and sharing. And food – when prepared by their parents – is a symbol of love. To be excluded from certain kinds of food, as many allergic children are, can feel deep down like an unfair punishment – a feeling which not only causes stress but which may affect children's behaviour too.

Case Study
Jason

In the Introduction we heard the story of Jason, aged 11, who has a severe allergy to brazil nuts, as well as some other nuts, cats and certain washing powders.

Jason knows that he has a serious, potentially life-threatening condition. He accepts that he has to be careful and – unless he can check the ingredients – always says a polite 'No thank you' when people other than his family offer him food. He doesn't make a fuss about his allergies, but there is no doubt that they make his life complicated, and that he feels he is missing out on certain pleasures in life:

'Having allergies is quite annoying', says Jason. 'I miss out on things; food mostly, especially chocolates. I have to check the labels on everything I eat. When I go to my friends' birthday parties my mum makes me a special lunch box so that I won't eat anything with nuts in by mistake. It is a pain having to look on the box to see what the ingredients are – but having an allergic reaction is even more annoying! Mostly I find it embarrassing when my lips and face swell up. It is quite scarey too when I get a bad reaction because then I find it hard to breathe. But I don't think about it a lot. One of my best friends has asthma attacks; another one of my friends is allergic to milk and so he has to have soya products all the time. I know I'm not the only one with allergies!'

So how can you as a parent help your child to acknowledge and come to terms with how he feels about having an allergy or an intolerance? As ever, communication is vital. If you had allergies as a child (or still do) try talking with your child about how it felt (feels) for you and what difference it has made to your life. This should help your child to express his own feelings, while also helping you to appraise yours; it will bring you closer, too.

Do give your child a chance to tell you about any bad or miserable feelings he may have. It is important to acknowledge these, they are very real; then, look on the bright side and end the conversation on a positive note.

It is also important for children to feel safe in the knowledge that you, their parents, know how to take care of them. Having an asthma attack for instance can be very scary for a child: it can be very scarey for you to, but if you are well prepared and well informed you will be able to stay calm and help your child to stay calm too.

Having an allergy can be damaging for your child's confidence in subtle ways that you may not at first notice, because you live with him all the time. Perhaps he may be reluctant to take part in sports at school: is this because he worries about having an asthma attack? Or because he doesn't want to change his clothes in case his classmates see his skin condition? Are other children teasing, even bullying him, at school or in social groups?

If so, you may need to take some strong action to boost your child's morale and self-esteem. Spend time with him, showing him that you enjoy his company. Tell him as often as you can that he is well loved and praise his achievements to all and sundry – in his earshot. Organize outings, events, parties which are the envy of all of his schoolmates. Encourage him to invite friends home after school and make sure they have a slap up meal and plenty of fun.

Even young children (from about seven years upwards) can benefit from techniques like yoga and meditation which can be a tremendous boost to calmness and self-esteem. This could become very special for you and your child to do together, bringing you closer and helping you both to deal with the stresses of having allergies and/or intolerances in the family.

Try also to strike a balance between getting your child the treatment he needs and helping him to feel that he is a basically healthy person. The right amount of loving attention – including medicines or remedies – can be very therapeutic. Too much and there is a risk that he will see himself as a sick person, which won't help him to get better.

Involving your child in endless rounds of clinic visits with the waiting area crowded with unwell people can be a depressing experience and he is bound to think: 'Am I like that?' So try whenever possible to organize his treatments from home by telephone. Many doctors will gladly consult with you or answer queries on the telephone, while complementary practitioners too are often happy to work with you on this basis.

Finally, when it comes to the business of healing, there is no substitute for a loving touch and children in particular are sensitive to this. Many conventional doctors are sceptical about the benefits of complementary therapies, such as aromatherapy or flower remedies, arguing that their effect is 'all in the mind'. This may be so, but the mind is a very powerful influence in health, and if your child knows that you love him and are doing your best to make him feel better, feel better he will.

YOUR FEELINGS

Parents' feelings about their children's problems are likely to be profound, complex and influential. Your feelings are bound to affect your child's feelings – and vice versa. Your stress can all too easily become his stress, making his allergies worse, and so the difficulties spiral. Becoming aware of how you feel, acknowledging and giving space to your feelings, and then being as positive as possible, is as important for you as it is for your child.

Most parents remember all too clearly how the whole business began: that anxious process of wondering whether their child has an allergy such as asthma, taking him to the doctor for tests and waiting for a diagnosis. And the fact that asthma is so widespread makes the ordeal of hearing the news no less traumatic.

The first blow: hearing the news

For Sarah, it all began when her daughter Toni was nine. After a series of winter colds Toni woke up one morning, struggling for breath. 'I took her to our family doctor', says Sarah, 'and he got her to blow into a peak flow meter and her reading turned out to be only one third of what it should have been.' Toni went home with prescriptions for 'preventer' and 'reliever' medicines (see Chapter four), and with the knowledge that there had been a significant change in her life. 'It is painful, as a mother', says Sarah, 'to hear your child diagnosed with some-thing which could affect her for the rest of her life.'

It is the long-term nature of an allergy like asthma and the prospect of perhaps having to take drugs every day, forever, which can be so difficult for parents to accept. But for Toni, so far, life goes on much as before – except that she has to try to remember to take her medicines. Today's children see asthma as no big deal. Says Toni: 'There are three other children in my class who have asthma, and some of them have it really badly, much worse than me.'

A whole family affair

Any severe allergy or intolerance can have a major emotional impact not just on the child affected, but on the whole family, parents and siblings, too. Some of the important things in life, such as sleep and food, are suddenly under threat. Parents can get worried and worn out, all their attention focused on one child. No matter how sympathetic his brothers and sisters may be, deep down there are bound to be tensions and resentments.

Nicky, now aged 16 years, has asthma and eczema. 'The asthma was part of a severe allergic reaction to milk which first showed up when she was three years old' says her mother Shelley. 'She was on Ventolin syrup from the age of three, but her first hospital admission for an asthma attack was at the age of eight.' Nicky has spent much of her young life learning to manage her asthma, which at times has been frighteningly severe. 'It has been grim,' admits Shelley. 'We have to take her in to hospital quite regularly. And every time she goes to hospital the whole family is affected. It is a strain on all of us. Her brothers and sisters all react in their own different ways. Her younger brother is always badly behaved when she goes to hospital, whereas for me there is the constant dilemma of "shall

I call the doctor, or the ambulance? Is she bad enough to take to hospital?"'

Always on the alert

A severe allergy, especially one which carries the risk of an anaphylactic reaction, also means that parents are constantly on the lookout for sources of trouble – which may come from the most unexpected quarters. For Sally, Jason's mother, the knowledge that her son is so vulnerable to any contact with nuts can mean rethinking everyday actions – like giving a child a kiss – that most parents take for granted:

'If I've been eating nuts I can't even kiss him in case it causes a reaction. If his father eats nuts he won't go near Jason either. At school last Christmas someone brought in a bag of brazil nuts for the class party. I asked for them to be taken out of the classroom; after all, they are potentially fatal for Jason. Every time I go shopping now I check to make sure that nothing I buy contains nuts. A lot of foods do have nut products, so the result is that we have mainly fruit, vegetables and soya products. We have to avoid yogurts and certain chocolate bars and biscuits. But it's not an issue at home; his sisters don't seem to mind.'

Making a fuss

Convincing other people of the dangers of a severe reaction can be quite a problem for parents of children with allergies and/or intolerances. Laura, now a teenager, has had asthma since she was a toddler and her mother has at times had difficulty explaining to other people that her daughter was at risk: 'When she went to play at other children's houses I'm sure that their parents thought I was just fussing. They could see a perfectly healthy-looking child, and I was trying to explain to them about the dangers of her asthma. It was hard to part with her sometimes, knowing that people might not be taking my warnings seriously.'

Those guilty feelings

On top of all this there is often guilt – that scourge of all mothers – as to *why* their child has developed allergies in the first place. This is not a rational feeling, but it is nonetheless real. As Ann, George's mother, puts it: 'I still feel awful that I didn't put it right when he was a little baby. I am still more anxious about him than I am about my younger children, although that has eased off as he has grown older.' Sometimes the guilt, mixed with regret, extends to the rest of the family. 'George's allergy problem has had an impact on the whole family,' says Ann. 'His younger sister certainly got ignored a bit because we were so preoccupied with George and getting him better. It has been a long, hard haul. It's amazing how many people still don't know that the cause of their children's health problems might be allergy, but when you've got a screaming baby, the last place you can settle down to do some research is your local library! When I see other mothers now who are wondering if their child might be allergic and if they ought to cut out certain foods, I always say – "Just try it!"

An antidote to guilt?
Deep down in almost every parents' psyche is the nagging feeling that if only they had done something more their child might not have this problem. This is why it may help to know that doing something *less* may actually be a good idea. Namely, keeping your child clean!

When the Institute of Child Health in the UK looked at asthma and hygiene, they came up with some interesting statistics:

- Small children who bathe every day and wash their hands more than five times a day are 25 per cent more likely to have asthma than those who don't.

- 46 per cent of children 'usually' washed their hands
  before every meal, but only 16 per cent washed their
  hands before every meal, while 9 per cent occasionally did
  and 2 per cent never did.

This research has raised the issue of whether higher modern
standards of hygeine mean that children are coming into
contact with less dirt and therefore fewer infections. Just
as mass vaccination programmes are cutting down on the
number of infections children experience, so may our habits
of cleanliness be contributing to the rise in children's
allergies.

HEALTH AND RELAXATION FOR YOU

Parents who have children with ailments of any kind are subject
to a form of stress which rarely eases off completely. Allergies
and/or intolerances in the family, however mild or severe, bring
their own particular pressures.

It's entirely understandable that parents of children with
potentially fatal allergies will at times suffer extreme anxiety.
Parents of children with long-term, low-level symptoms will also
have been through many months, even years, of worry. And
parents of children whose allergies make them hyperactive are
often totally exhausted.

But the very nature of being a parent means that your energies
tend to be focused on your child rather on yourself. Most of us
don't ever have to throw ourselves under a bus to save our
child, but the same fundamental instinct is there in our day-to-
day care and attention. The more children we have – the more
thinly spread we are, giving as much as we can – often without
anyone else to take care of *us*. Inevitably, our energies, physical
and emotional, become depleted. If our children also have
allergies and/or intolerances, then the demand made upon us
are even greater.

In many other cultures, and at other times in history, there would probably have been sisters, grandmothers, in-laws, neighbours to help the mother out in times of trouble. As the African saying goes, it takes a village to raise a child. Sadly these days, one or two parents are expected to have all the human resources of the traditional village. No wonder we get stressed and worn out.

This is why looking after yourself is crucial. For a start, you deserve it; second if you don't look after yourself, sooner or later *you* are likely to get ill, and then who will give your child the care and attention that he needs? So,

Be sensible and . . .
- Make sure you get plenty of exercise, gentle or vigorous, according to your own fitness level. Even 20 minutes a day will help you to withstand everyday pressures and can help you avoid a build-up of stress. Remember that exercise doesn't have to mean getting sweaty and exhausted. Holistic forms of exercise such as yoga and t'ai chi can help you keep fit physically, as well as mentally and emotionally, without making you feel tired.
- Eat well, choosing fresh foods whenever possible (and preferably certified organic), eating five portions of fruit and vegetables daily (a portion fits into the palm of your hand).
- Drink chamomile tea (especially the organically cultivated kind), rather than tea or coffee to help you to relax at bedtime.
- Start your day with a bowl of organic, whole-oat porridge. Too many of us are so busy looking after children and getting them off to school in the morning that we neglect to give ourselves a decent breakfast. Unrefined oats provide not only instant energy, but slow-release energy to keep you going all morning. Some complementary practitioners believe they also have a calming effect on your system, which may benefit your heart and encourage healthy circulation by helping to prevent a build-up of cholesterol.
- Avoid excessive alcohol consumption; this can make you seriously depressed, raise your blood pressure and disrupt your much-needed sleep. And don't smoke: cigarettes may seem to offer a moment of relaxation, but in fact they are

full of poisons which can do your body nothing but harm –
let alone the implications smoking has for asthma and other
problems.

- Try to get plenty of sleep. A modicum of exercise during the
  day, going to bed in good time and a hot drink such as
  chamomile tea at bedtime can help you to have a restful
  night.
- Treat yourself to a soothing aromatherapy massage from time
  to time, or try one of the other relaxing complementary
  therapies, such as reflexology. These will not only help you
  to relax and feel good, but will boost your immune system,
  helping to maintain your health and well-being.
- Get a trusted babysitter, go out, see friends and – the best
  medicine – have a laugh!

Chapter Four

Conventional Treatments

▥ THE FIRST STEP

For most parents, the first step in getting treatment for a child with suspected allergy or intolerance is the family doctor. If your doctor agrees that allergy is the root of the problem, you may be referred to an allergy specialist, or allergist. However, there are not many allergists around, so your child may be referred to another kind of specialist, depending on his symptoms.

The most commonly recognized children's allergies are asthma, eczema and hayfever and, for these, conventional medicine has a range of drug treatments to offer. In the case of food allergy and intolerance, however, the situation is less clear because, as we have seen, substances that can cause one set of symptoms in one person can cause different symptoms in another.

So, because symptoms of food allergy and intolerance do not follow a recognizable pattern, doctors can overlook them, especially if they do not involve the classic IgE reaction. To complicate matters further, the symptoms are often mistaken for everyday ailments because they often show up as headaches, or tummy pains, complaints which don't normally merit medical attention.

The big exception to this general rule is anaphylactic shock (see p.49). Not only is this instantly recognizable as a severe allergic reaction, with a (usually) identifiable trigger, but doctors take this very seriously indeed as a potentially life-threatening condition. You should never underestimate the dangers of ana-phylaxsis and conventional medicine has saved many lives with its emergency treatments with drugs such as adrenaline (epinephrine).

Conventional medicine has no 'cure' for allergy or intolerance (although immunotherapy can help sufferers with severe symp-toms – see below). Progress is being made, however, in tracking down the gene which may make children susceptible to asthma; doctors hope this may lead to a cure in the future. Researchers are also trying to develop a 'vaccine' which they hope will block allergic reactions to peanuts and other foods. In the meantime there are many drug treatments which can allieviate symptoms.

The good news for parents is that most children grow out of their allergies without treatment. By the age of four years, more than two-thirds of children affected by allergy no longer suffer and by aged two, four in five infants allergic to milk will have overcome the allergy. Around one-third of children grow out of their asthma in their teens, while for another third, the symp-toms improve considerably or there are longer stretches between attacks.

However, until that time – or if your child is experiencing distressing symptoms – it is important to see your family doctor, not only to discuss treatments but to exclude other conditions which you may have mistaken for allergy or intolerance. Remember, too, that some of these conditions can be extremely dangerous – even fatal – and others can, in the long term, cause permanent damage to health. Even if you tend to prefer self-help and complementary therapies, it is worth seeing your doctor for a diagnosis, and to find out the options offered by conven-tional medicine.

TESTING FOR ALLERGIES

As allergies have become increasingly common in the past 30 years, there has been a proliferation of diagnostic tests. Most doctors will not test for food allergies, but you may be referred to an allergy specialist. However, only a minority of these believe that food can cause allergy and intolerance.

Allergy specialists (allergists) may offer the RAST or ELISA tests outlined below. Some may know of and have access to the ALCAT and FACT methods of testing.

Two tests used routinely:
- **The skin prick test** This involves pricking the skin and placing solutions of suspected allergens on it. If your child is allergic to that particular substance, an inflamed weal will form on her skin at the site of testing within about 15 minutes. The bigger and more inflamed the weal, the more sensitive your child is likely to be to that substance.

  This test can be useful for children who react to inhaled allergens, but is less useful when it comes to food allergies.
- **RAST (the radioallergosorbent test)** This is a blood test in which a sample of blood is mixed with the suspected allergen. The antibody response is then measured. This test only measures the IgE reaction – i.e. of one particular immunoglobulin. However, some experts believe that other immunoglobulins and chemicals involved in certain allergies, especially food allergies, will not be picked up by RAST.

Case Study
A testing experience . . .

Luke's mother took him to their family doctor after he reacted violently to something he had eaten. He had sickness, weals and stomach cramps. 'Our doctor recommended the RAST blood test and we were referred to a paediatrician at our local hospital who is an allergy specialist. Luke was very little and he was very worried about having the needles in the back of his hand, and by the idea of having his blood taken. But the specialist was very kind and put special "magic" (local anaesthetic) cream on his hand first. We had to wait a couple of weeks for the RAST test result. I was really worried that Luke might be very allergic to peanuts which are in a lot of different foods. But the test told us that he scored three for brazil nuts (the highest level of reaction); two for hazelnuts; one for walnuts and peanuts and zero for almonds. That means he has a very serious, potentially fatal reaction to brazil nuts.'

More sophisticated blood tests have been designed to pick up a wider range of potential allergens, but these are not commonly available. They include:

- ELISA **(Enzyme Linked ImmunoSorbent Assay)** This is a blood test which detects IgG and IgA reactions.
- ALCAT **(Antigen, Leucocyte Cellular Antibody Test)** This is a cytotoxic test designed to measure the activity of white blood cells.
- FACT **(Food Allergy Cellular Test)** This blood test is considered to be 'state of the art' by leading complementary practitioners. It is not widely available but you can ask your doctor to send a blood sample for testing at private laboratories (see Useful Addresses).

For more details about FACT see Chapter five.

Testing by the elimination diet

If you think your child's allergic reaction is being caused by food, one common method for tracing the allergens involved is the elimination or exclusion diet. Any elimination diet for children should always be supervised by an allergy specialist or qualified nutritionist.

Under this regimen your child is to eat from only a limited selection of foods which have been proved to be rarely allergenic – such as lamb, pears, rice, turkey and parsnips. New foods are gradually re-introduced into the diet one at a time, and their effect monitored to see whether they provoke a reaction. New foods are re-introduced at three-day intervals, because it can take up to 72 hours before a reaction is seen in your child's body.

This makes the elimination diet not only slow and laborious, but difficult for many children to follow in practical terms. It can be very hard to explain – especially to a young child – that she can go to a friend's party but not eat the party food! It can also be tough for parents to shop for and cook such a restricted diet while keeping the rest of the family happy. But remember that this is the most effective way to reduce or get rid of symptoms.

■ TREATMENTS

Treatments for allergies depend very much on the type of allergy and/or intolerance and the symptoms shown. The best and safest 'treatment' for allergy and intolerance is simply to *avoid the allergen which is causing the problem*. This is only possible once you know what that allergen is – and for many children there are more than one. Sometimes, though, it is simply impossible to avoid an allergen, such as pollen, although you can take steps to reduce your child's exposure.

■ Asthma

The number of children with asthma in the Western world has been spiraling upwards in recent decades, with at least one in seven schoolchildren diagnosed with asthma in the UK alone and even higher numbers in some other countries.

Doctors still don't understand fully the causes of asthma, but its symptoms include inflammation and narrowing of the airways which, together with the production of thick mucus, makes it difficult to breathe. Asthma may be triggered by a range of substances, including dust, animal dander, cigarette smoke, traffic fumes; it may also be brought on by flu or cold air – and stress.

Orthodox medical opinion is divided as to whether asthma can be triggered by eating certain foods, although complementary practitioners argue that they have good evidence that it can.

Asthma: the major culprits:

- Dairy products
- Seafood
- Yeast
- Nuts

If you think your child is allergic to particular foods, the best thing to is avoid them – regardless of whether you have medical 'proof' or not. (See elimination diets p.40.)

You know your child better than anyone, so you can help your doctor by compiling a list of symptoms along with any suspected triggers and when symptoms occur.

Common symptoms to look out for:

- Long-lasting cough, often worse at night and after exercise
- Wheezing
- Shortness of breath
- Chest tightness

Case Study
Tanya, aged 10

'When I get asthma I have a really tight chest, like I'm being squashed. It's really hard to breathe and I feel tired, breathless and wheezy. It can happen at any time of day, but it's worst when I've been running about a lot. It's very annoying.'

Marion, mother of Laura, now in her teens:

'It was very hard to pin down the triggers of Laura's asthma.

It could have been pollen; it could have been dust mites or mould spore – we never really knew. But too much excitement certainly set her off. Year after year when she was little, Laura missed her own birthday parties – we simply had to cancel them at the last minute because she became so breathless. She missed out on family walks too because cold winds would sometimes trigger her asthma – but at other times they wouldn't. It was very hard to predict. Fortunately, once she reached her teens, her symptoms disappeared.'

Seeing your doctor

Your doctor will ask if there is a family history of asthma or related atopic conditions such as eczema and hayfever. In an older child (aged six, or more), your doctor may take a series of peak flow meter readings using a small hand-held meter to show how fast air is leaving the lungs when your child exhales; this indicates whether her airways are narrowed.

'Relievers' and 'preventers'

There are basically two types of asthma treatments commonly used today. The first type, 'relievers' or bronchodilators, relax the muscles around the airways when a 'trigger' hits them and they constrict. Relievers can be taken as a rescue when your child feels symptoms coming on, or when she expects them to come on – as when taking exercise.

'Relievers' are usually taken from an inhaler and they include the drugs salbutamol (known by the trade names of Ventolin, Salbulin or Aerolin) and terbutaline (Bricanyl or Brethine). There are also longer-lasting relievers available for people with more severe asthma, which can be taken from an inhaler or in tablet form.

The reliever drugs act in a similar manner to adrenaline (epinephrine), the substance our bodies naturally produce to get ready for action (sometimes called the 'fight or flight' chemical). Adrenaline not only makes the heart beat faster, it also opens the airways.

Reliever medicines, especially when taken in high doses, can have unwanted side-effects, such as shaking hands, nausea and palpitations, but doctors say that although these may be unpleasant they are not dangerous.

Many complementary practitioners argue that in fact these medicines make the asthma worse in the long term (see Chapter five). Some medical professionals also believe that the long-term use of drugs to manage allergies can have a detrimental effect on the immune system.

'Preventers' are medicines designed to treat inflammation of the airways in order to stop asthma symptoms from appearing when your child meets a 'trigger'. They have to be used regularly. Children who need preventers are likely to be given a non-steroid drug such as sodium cromoglycate (cromolyn sodium) known as Intal. This protects against allergic triggers as well as exercise-induced asthma and is the first line of treatment for children with allergic asthma. If sodium cromoglycate doesn't work, however, children are sometimes prescribed one of the inhaled steroid drugs (such as beclomethasone or budesonide) more usually given to adults. Preventers may have side-effects which can include headache, cough, palpitations, mild tremor and mouth dryness.

In most cases, children with asthma take their medication by inhalation, but for children who are too young to master the inhalation technique, or who are fearful of the 'spacers' and/or masks provided to assist inhalation in young children, pills and syrups are available. However, as these drugs have to go through the child's bloodstream to reach the lungs, they do not work as quickly as inhaled medication. They also have to be given in a higher dose, increasing the risk of unwanted side-effects.

The majority of children with asthma have only mild-to-moderate symptoms which can be managed with low-dose inhaled steroids with a low-risk of side-effects. Similarly, occasional courses of steroid tablets or syrup to bring an asthma attack under control appears to carry minimal risk.

Emergency action: dealing with an asthma attack
Although asthma is far from rare, it can still be very dangerous, as Marion, Laura's mother, recalls:

'We couldn't hear Laura wheezing so we thought that she was all right – until we saw that she had gone blue. She couldn't even speak because so little air was going in and out of her lungs. We called our doctor, but if we had known how close she was to slipping into unconsciousness, we would have called an ambulance too.'

An asthma attack is defined as when the reliever treament is not rescuing the sufferer from breathing difficulties after the first 5–10 minutes of taking it. In their booklet 'Take Control of Asthma' the UK National Asthma Campaign suggests taking the following steps should your child have an asthma attack:

- She should take the reliever again after 5 to 10 minutes.
- Help her to stay calm: she needs to relax as much as her breathing will allow.
- Encourage her to sit up in a position which she finds comfortable, with her hands on her knees to help support her back.
- Encourage her to slow down her breathing if possible.
- If the reliever is still not working – or you notice two or more of the following danger signs – call an ambulance/paramedics.

Danger signs: get your child immediately to hospital if you notice TWO OR MORE of these warning signs:

1 Breathing is twenty times a minute or more
2 Pulse rate is over 100 beats per minute
3 Speaking is very difficult
4 There is dizziness or fainting
5 There is blueness around the lips

▉ ECZEMA

This skin condition is often an allergic response, in which case it is known as atopic dermatitis. This can manifest as a dry, itchy inflammation of the skin, and it can make life an utter misery for children – and their parents, too. Almost one in five children will experience eczema at some time, and the numbers are increasing. Eczema can cause intolerable itching, keeping children and parents awake at night, and in extreme cases hospitalization may be necessary. It is most common in families with a history of allergies including asthma and hayfever.

▉ Diagnosis and treatment

Your doctor will ask if there is a history of allergies in your family. She will also inspect your child's rash which often appears behind the knees, in the creases of the elbows, in the groin and on the cheeks.

Orthodox medical treatment involves suppressing the symptoms (rather than addressing the causes) of eczema. These are usually in the form of creams which contain corticosteriod drugs (topical steroid creams), combined with emollient creams and lotions to moisturize your child's skin. Topical steroids work by controlling and damping down inflammation in the skin. They alleviate the itching of eczema, so that children will be less inclined to scratch – in turn giving the skin a chance to heal.

Some corticosteroid medication (such as prednisolone and prednisone) may be given orally, although some doctors will avoid prescribing them because of the risk of side-effects. Steroids can be very effective in the short term, but the more you use them, the less effective they may become in the long term, and the side-effects may become unacceptable.

Coal-tar pastes and ointments have been used for skin inflammation for many years and they remain an effective form of treatment. Unfortunately, they are messy, smell unpleasant and may stain clothes and bedlinen. They are usually applied to children at bedtime under bandages, or applied in the form of pre-impregnanted bandages which are easier to use. The bandages have the added advantage of preventing children from scratching their skin during the night.

Occasionally, doctors will also prescribe:

- Antibiotics if the eczema becomes infected.
- Antihistamine tablets although these can cause drowsiness or sometimes hyperactivity.
- Ultraviolet light (UVA) treatment in combination with the drug psoralen is known as PUVA, and although this is not widely available, it can be effective for children or adolescents who have suffered from eczema for many years.

HAYFEVER

Hayfever, or allergic rhinitis, is one of the most common allergies. Around one in ten of the population of the UK for example is affected; boys most commonly between the ages of 5 and 15, girls between 15 and 20 years. Hayfever is particularly common amongst people who already have asthma. The good news is that in half of the sufferers hayfever simply disappears – often after a particularly bad year. Even for those who don't get a reprieve, the symptoms tend to wear off with age as the immune response becomes less strong.

As with eczema, this is not a life-threatening condition but the symptoms can be extremely distressing. Chiefly caused by pollen and mould spores, a bad case of hayfever is rather like having a terrible cold, coupled with extreme irritation of the eyes and nose. Constant sneezing and watering eyes add to the misery, and children with hayfever are likely to feel very tired too. Symptoms are usually at their worst in June, just when children want to be outside enjoying the fresh air and summer sunshine. Hayfever – with all the mucus produced – may also cause a degree of deafness in young children, which may go unrecognized.

■ Treatments

Some doctors favour the new generation of one-dose antihistamine tablets which have no sedative side-effects but which act on the whole body. Others prefer local, targeted treatments which include nasal corticosteroids and nasal antihistamines for a very blocked nose, or eye drops containing antihistamine and decongestant for very puffy eyes. Most doctors consider preventive eye and nose drops made from sodium cromoglycate to be safe and effective, even for young children.

Desensitizing injections (see p.50) may be considered by your doctor if your child has very severe hayfever. However, these have to be taken all year round and mean regular visits to the hospital or clinic. Since most children hate needles and injections, this should only be considered as a last resort.

Now that the trigger for hayfever has been identified as part of a protein called profilin, a new treatment for the condition may eventually be forthcoming.

> **Environmental allergies**
> Although there are varying levels of scepticism among orthodox doctors about environmental allergies, it is theoretically possible that any substance can cause an allergy. The most common suspects in our environment include:
>
> * Pollen
> * Dust mite faeces
> * Moulds
> * Feathers
> * Nickel
> * Latex
> * Dander of furry animals

Scientific research is now concentrating on developing vaccines to particular allergens, but in the meantime, avoidance is widely considered the best policy (once the trigger has been identified).

For more details on how to prevent your child from suffering allergic symptoms at home, see p.20.

FOOD ALLERGIES AND SENSITIVITIES

Received medical wisdom divides food sensitivity into two categories: food allergy and food intolerance. In food allergy the reaction to certain food is often severe, with vomiting, rashes, eczema, asthma, or even anaphylactic shock. This latter occurs very soon – sometimes immediately – after the allergen is eaten.

The other type of sensitivity is known as food intolerance. This produces a less acute and much slower reaction, and while complementary practitioners believe it to be very common, orthodox doctors are more sceptical. Intolerance is often triggered by foods that are eaten often, such as wheat or dairy products. They are often foods that the sufferer craves and eating them satisfies the craving but leads to other problems. Avoiding the offending food for some months can usually alleviate food intolerance, and after a while, the food can often be re-introduced without causing problems.

Unfortunately, little medical help is available for food allergies and sensitivity. However, the very severe reaction of anaphylaxis requires immediate medical attention.

ANAPHYLAXIS

Anaphylaxsis can be triggered by a variety of allergens, the most common of which are foods (especially peanuts, nuts, eggs, cow's milk, shellfish); certain drugs, such as penicillin; the venom of stinging insects (such as bees, wasps and hornets); latex and paint.

On contact with the allergen, the body's cells release huge quantities of histamine which causes the blood vessels to swell suddenly. This often affects the lungs, throat and mouth, causing breathing difficulties that can be life threatening. The skin also becomes flushed and hives may appear. Blood vessels begin to leak causing a dramatic drop in blood pressure. The sufferer often passes out.

If your child is at risk of anaphylaxsis, your doctor will prescribe medication for use in the event of an allergic reaction. This may include an injection of adrenaline (epinephrine). The adrenaline injections that are most commonly prescribed are the EpiPen, the Anapen and the Min-I-Jet. These devices are preloaded and very simple to administer. Antihistamines and hydrocortisone may also be given. For more information see Useful Addresses.

Desensitization
Desensitization or 'immunotherapy' is a treatment offered by some allergy clinics for people with hayfever or eczema who react to inhaled allergens. This treatment has been around for many years, although doubts about its safety following a number of deaths have meant that it is still not widely available.

Desensitization works on the theory that if you inject the body with minute amounts of whatever is causing the allergic reaction, gradually increasing the doses, the body will build up a resistance and restore tolerance to those allergens.

First, a blood test establishes the offending allergen. Then, treatment is given at intervals. This treatment is successful for some people.

Enzyme potentiated desensitization is a more sophisticated form of desensitization which is becoming more widely available. It can help people with food intolerance problems as well as other allergies. It too involves a blood test to establish the nature of the allergens, followed by a course of injections. It differs technically from standard desensitization techniques in that the compound glucuronidase is attached to the injected allergen.

▪ SIDE-EFFECTS OF DRUG TREATMENTS

Many parents of children with allergies have understandable anxieties that conventional drug treatments for allergies may have unwanted – or even dangerous – side-effects. It is true that most drugs have some side-effects, however, adverse reactions to drugs for allergies are rare, and in most cases the risk of side-effects is very small. Your doctor should alert you to any risks involved with prescribed medication, as well as monitoring your child carefully throughout her treatment.

In asthma treatment, for example, bronchodilators have been associated with increased heart rate, trembling and headaches, while some medical professionals have expressed concerns that overuse of relievers may make asthma symptoms worse. Others fear that the long-term use of drugs to manage allergies may have a detrimental effect on the immune system, leaving us more susceptible to viral and other infections.

For most parents though, the greatest anxiety is caused by putting children on steroid drugs from a young age. Steroids have had a bad press in recent years, partly because they have been (wrongly) associated with the drugs sometimes taken illegally by athletes, and partly because of the long list of side-effects they may cause. These include lowered immunity, growth retardation, diabetes, glaucoma and osteoporosis. High doses for extended periods can also adversely affect the functioning of the adrenal glands. Steroids applied topically (as a cream, say, as for eczema) may also cause thinning of the skin over a long period.

Yet despite these worrying side-effects, it is important not to lose sight of the fact that children are put on this kind of medication to treat symptoms which are likely to be far more dangerous. It is children with severe asthma who need high or prolonged doses of these drugs. Their doctors will be well aware of the risks of side-effects and will reduce their medication wherever possible.

Most children have mild or moderate asthma which can be controlled with low-dose inhaled steroids – with a very low risk of side-effects. Occasional courses of steroid tablets or syrup to bring an asthma attack under control also have few long-term health risks. If you do suspect that your child's treatment is causing problems, or that her immune system is suffering (i.e. if she has repeated viral or other infections), you should consult your doctor.

There may be other ways in which you can help your child (avoiding the allergens for instance) so that the dosage of her drugs can be lowered. You can also help her to stay well while reducing the risk of side-effects from drugs by:

- Making sure your child eats a healthy, balanced, diet where the foodstuffs resemble their original state as much as possible – i.e. avoid convenience and processed food as much as you can. Organic produce is best. It costs a little more but is packed full of immune boosting nutrients.
- Seeing a complementary therapist who can help improve your child's general health in order to fight both the allergy symptoms and the effects of drug treatment. By using complementary therapies it may also be possible to reduce your child's medication, or even to stop it altogether.

The next chapter looks at those complementary therapies which have most to offer children with allergies.

Chapter Five

Complementary Therapies

If you have already tried the conventional medical approach to tackling your child's allergy, but without the success you hoped for, it may be worth considering the complementary therapies. Indeed, many complementary practitioners would argue that it is better to try complementary methods *before* trying orthodox medication which could complicate your child's health problems further.

Complementary therapies are becoming increasingly popular in the West. There are several reasons for this, but one is that they do not involve taking prescription drugs – which may have unwanted side-effects, especially in young children. Another major plus for complementary therapies is that your practitioner will take plenty of time to assess and treat your child, not just as a set of symptoms, but as a whole person.

This aspect of complementary medicine is often healing in itself. For as all parents know, giving a child (especially a young child) plenty of sympathy and attention can have a genuinely therapeutic effect – which is why parents cuddle a child who has taken a tumble, rub the bruised knee or 'kiss it better'. Human care and contact can make all the difference to your child's ability to put up with pain and make a good recovery.

The holistic approach also means that a complementary practitioner will not concentrate solely on your child's allergies, but will work towards building up his health and immunity in general. For this reason we will look at the complementary therapies and remedies which are most effective for allergies and intolerances as a whole, rather than as a set of symptoms (such as eczema or asthma) as we did in the last chapter. This can bring wide benefits, such as being better able to fight off infections and the effects of pollution on the body.

Many doctors now accept that complementary therapies can help with problems like allergy and intolerance, and give their support to patients who want to try this route. In Britain, 40 per cent of family doctors now offer access to holistic services and one in four people have used complementary medicine. In the USA, the figure is even higher with one in three Americans using some form of complementary medicine.

Of course, complementary medicine has its opponents and the media backlash against its popularity has been particularly strong in recent years. Its critics say that complementary therapies are not proven to be safe and effective in the same way as modern drugs. However, there are thousands of studies in many languages – usually ignored by Western doctors – which testify to the effectiveness of complementary treatments.

There is also a case to be argued that orthodox methods used for testing drugs (such as the double-blind trial in which neither doctor nor patient knows whether they are receiving the active drug or a placebo) are not appropriate for many complementary therapies. Acupuncture for instance cannot be 'proven' to be effective through double-blind studies – but then neither can modern surgery!

■ CHOOSING A THERAPIST

Allergy and intolerance can be a serious threat to your child's health and it is important that you satisfy yourself that the therapist you have chosen is a good one. Most complementary therapies now have a regulatory body that sets standards of training and qualifications, provides insurance and ensures that members work to a code of ethics. These bodies can provide you with a register of practitioners (which should be updated annually) who practise in your area. You will find a list of regulatory bodies in the Useful Addresses section at the end of this book.

Taking the following steps will help ensure that your child receives the best complementary health care:

- If you are considering using a complementary therapy, do discuss this with your family doctor first. She may also be able to recommend you to a local practitioner she has worked with or referred to before. If not, see below.
- Ask friends and acquaintances who have used complementary therapies to recommend a practitioner.
- If you have no leads from either of these sources, approach the self-regulating body and ask for their register of practitioners. You could also ask if any of their members specialize in treating children with allergies.
- Contact a local complementary clinic (rather like a group medical practice) rather than an individual practitioner (on the basis that those who work within a group come under more scrutiny by their peers than lone practitioners!).
- Visit your practioner – and trust your instincts. He may be technically very expert, but if you or child doesn't feel comfortable with him this will compromise the success of the treatment. So if you don't like him, go elsewhere!

Once you have found a complementary therapist and your child has started receiving treatment, *do not suddenly stop taking conventional medication.* Ideally, you should inform your doctor that your child is seeing a complementary therapist (and vice versa) so that both can work together to alleviate your child's allergies.

In reality, conventional health professionals and complementary therapists tend to be suspicious of one another and cooperation is the exception rather than the rule.

If all goes well with your child's complementary treatment, however, you will begin to see an improvement in his symptoms with a corresponding drop in his need for medication – and an improvement in your family doctor's appreciation of complementary therapies! If, on the other hand, your doctor remains uncooperative, you have the right to change your doctor and to find someone who is more open to the practice of complementary therapies.

And a word of warning: do be wary of over-the-counter preparations, such as nutritional or mega-vitamin supplements, creams or herbal tablets. As we have seen, allergy and intolerance is very complex and each child's specific triggers will vary, as will their symptoms. You are better advised to spend your money on a well-qualified practitioner who will give you advice that is tailored specifically to your child.

Once complementary treatment is underway, monitor your child closely. There is often an 'acute' stage in which symptoms will get worse, but this should only last for a day or two and then your child should start to make real progress. This acute stage is not the time to give up on your chosen therapy; it is actually a sign that it is working! However, if symptoms do get steadily worse, contact your practitioner to discuss the situation. Do not feel pressurized to continue if you are unhappy with the treatment.

METHODS OF TESTING FOR ALLERGIES

Self-help tests

The best kind of self-help test for allergy (in complementary as well as in conventional medicine) is to avoid the suspected allergen. This could be an elimination diet, or it could mean staying away from cats, but the rationale is the same: if the symptoms of allergy disappear as a result of eliminating the suspected antigen, then you have a positive result.

Fact

In more complex cases, especially where there may be many allergens involved (see case history of Ruby, below), a FACT blood test is currently the most advanced allergy test available. Although FACT is not yet fully accepted by the orthodox medical world, it is the latest method of testing not only for IgE (as in conventional blood tests), but also for IgG4 (an immunoglobulin which is produced against certain foods and other allergens) and for leukotrienes (chemicals released by white blood cells that have recognized an invader).

FACT is available from private laboratories through complementary practitioners (see Useful Addresses).

Case Study
Ruby, aged eight, has been treated for allergies using nutritional therapy. Her mother outlines her progress:

When my daughter Ruby was two she began to suffer from a constantly blocked nose. It was particularly difficult at night-time as she couldn't breathe properly, which meant she couldn't sleep. She ended up having coughing fits almost every night which caused her to vomit, and only then could she sleep for two or three hours at a stretch. It was really terrible.

Our family doctor prescribed her antibiotics, but Ruby's

condition only got worse. She saw an allergy specialist who said that she was allergic to feathers, wool and dust and gave her medication, but again, it was no help. I went to so many doctors to try to find a solution, but we had no success.

After six years of this situation, I asked my friends about complementary practitioners and we went to see someone who specialized in allergies. He ran a FACT blood test on Ruby and discovered that she has very strong allergic responses to gluten, milk and eggs. That was four months ago and since then we have eliminated these from her diet and now her health is very good.

She has to avoid food like pasta, pizza, bread and cakes which is very hard for a little girl of eight. But I have started to bake bread especially for her, using a gluten-free baking mix. We also have to be careful with sliced meats like turkey and chicken because these often contain milk protein and wheat starch – so I read all the labels now.

I asked our practitioner if I could sometimes give her a little bit of gluten and he said we should only give it to her occasionally, if at all. I did give her one meal a day with a little gluten, but by the fourth day of this she started to get a blocked nose again.

It is tough for Ruby and she may have to be careful about what she eats for her whole life, but now at least we know what the problem is and we are very happy indeed with the great improvement in her health.

Gut permeability test

As we have seen, Leaky Gut Syndrome is a common cause of allergy (if not *the* most common cause), and if your practitioner suspects that this is problem in your child's case, he or she will suggest a Gut Permeability Test. This involves giving your child a solution to drink which contains many different sized molecules. His urine is then collected over a six-hour period and the size of the molecules present in the urine is measured. If there are very large molecules present – or if there are too many of one particular kind of molecule getting through the gut wall – then Leaky Gut Syndrome can be confirmed.

Bio-resonance

Some forms of complementary therapy also use their own methods of diagnosis to discover the cause of allergies. For instance, bio-resonance computers can be effective in identifying exactly what triggers your child's allergy or intolerance. Bio-resonance is described in more detail on p.68.

Popular – but unproven?
Other complementary techniques which are commonly used to test for allergies include the following:

- **Kinesiology** A phial containing a substance is placed on the child's abdomen, or the food itself is placed on the tongue (insist on phials if there is any risk of anaphylaxsis!). The practitioner then pushes against the patient's limb – usually the arm – to test for muscle weakness which is believed to reveal whether the substance is having a negative effect.
- **Hair analysis** A sample of hair is mixed with antibodies which react against selected substances. If those antibodies react – against wheat, for instance – this is believed to indicate a positive allergic response. The principle underlying hair analysis is that the body excretes noxious substances through the hair, so that the hair will show traces of whatever the body is allergic to.
- **Dowsing** A pendulum is held over a food while the practitioner is in contact with a patient.

There is little evidence that these methods are effective in detecting allergies, but it is possible that they may work for you.

WHICH THERAPY?

One of the problems often faced by people who want to try a complementary therapy is that there are so many of them, all apparently using different methods. So how do you decide which therapy is best for your child – and your child's allergies and/or intolerances? In practice – especially if you live in a rural area – you might find you don't have a great deal of choice: you may have a local homeopath or acupuncturist, but unless you are prepared to travel to the nearest city or big town, that could be it!

This next section of this Chapter covers those complementary therapies which take either a psychological approach, a medicinal approach – or what is becoming known as an 'energy medicine' approach (based on the Eastern philosophical belief that the energy flow through your body can be manipulated to improve health). Clearly, some of them are going to be more effective for your child's allergies or intolerances than others, and they appear in order of preference.

1. **Nutritional therapy** (with or without homeopathy) this should be the first line of complementary treatment for allergy or intolerance, involving changes in diet, backed up by specifically recommended nutritional supplements in conjunction with homeopathy.

If this line of treatment is not effective, the next best option is:

2. **Naturopathy** this is an umbrella term for a range of therapies which include hydrotherapy, nutritional advice, osteopathy, and relaxation and stress management. The naturopathic approach tackles Leaky Gut Syndrome (see Chapter two) by improving the condition of the bowel.

If you are not satisfied, try:

3. **Food remedies** in conjunction with Eastern medicine or herbal medicines (see p.65).

If your child still shows no sign of improvement, then try:

4. **Bio-resonance** treatments and/or **acupuncture** (see p.68).

If you still see no improvement in your child's allergies, it is worth considering:

5. **Psychological therapies** and **breathing techniques** (see p.72).

As a *support* to any of the above treatments, it may be worth your while to also try:

6. **Aromatherapy** (see p.75), **healing** (see p.76), **flower remedies** (see p.76)

NUTRITIONAL THERAPY

The use of food, vitamin, mineral and other nutrient supplements to cure and prevent disease is an increasingly scientific and complex field. Research supports the fact that a convenience- and junk-food diet can be associated not only with anti-social behaviour, but also with a wide range of everyday ailments. Moreover, an allergic reaction to certain foods can be the cause of any number of chronic ailments.

What to expect at a consultation

You will be asked to fill in a detailed questionnaire about your child. Once your therapist has studied his medical history, symptoms, diet and lifestyle, she may do a number of tests (such as blood or urine tests) to pinpoint any dietary problems, including digestive problems and allergies or intolerances to food, the environment and/or chemicals. Other practitioners prefer to rely on their own observations when making a diagnosis (bare in mind that most children hate giving blood samples).

Treatment programmes consist of nutritional education, a short-term diet tailored to your child and a course of supplements which may include vitamins, minerals or herbs. You may be advised generally on how to achieve the best possible balance in your child's diet with (for instance) 50 per cent of her food in the form of fruit and vegetables, 35 per cent grain and 15 per cent protein. You may be recommended to vary her intake of vegetables with deep green, light green, yellow, white and red vegetables in a 5:4:3:2:1 ratio.

This kind of diet can help to discourage the inflammatory process, to discourage the loss of bowel flora and the overgrowth of *Candida albicans*. It also ensures that there is plenty of fibre in your child's diet so that toxins cannot settle in and irritate his bowel. He may also be advised to drink half a pint of water for every foot of his height each day.

Some nutritional therapists may use food as medicine. Those trained in Eastern philosophies will regard food in terms of *Yin* (with the properties of fluid; fuelling the body) and *Yang* (with properties of heat; the spark that ignites the body's fuel).

■ HOMEOPATHY

The principle of this system is to 'treat like with like', and so patients are treated with tiny doses of substances that would cause the symptoms of their illness in a perfectly healthy person. This method is believed to stimulate the body's own healing processes – as opposed to treating symptoms alone which may bring only temporary relief.

There are hundreds of homeopathic remedies which are useful for treating allergies and/or interolerances, and homeopathy is widely regarded as a very safe form of therapy which is particularly effective for children. Much depends, however, (as with other treatments) on how you and your child manage when it comes to complicated issues such as diet and social life. Children today go to a lot of parties and eat a lot of highly processed foods. They may also have prescriptions for asthma medication or decongestants or antibiotics – which are likely to work against a course of homeopathy.

What to expect at a consultation

The homeopath will want to take your child's medical history, asking for details of his complaint and when it started. You may be asked to fill out quite a complicated form asking for all sorts of information – about personal quirks, emotions and even reactions to the weather – which you may not have been asked for before.

It is important to mention anything that could be a trigger for your child's allergy. For instance, if the allergy started a few weeks after you finished breastfeeding – and when you first gave your child cow's milk – then chances are that dairy products are triggering an allergic reaction.

As the tendency to allergy can be inherited, you may also be quizzed about your own and/or your partner's medical history, and whether there are any allergies in the family. Your child's past medical treatments may also be an issue: has he suffered any viral infections (these can trigger allergy), or experienced any changes in health after vaccinations?

The homeopath is also likely to suggest some kind of allergy test. Once you have established any substances or foods which trigger your child's allergies, you can discuss further treatment. Homeopathy offers various alternatives, ranging from desensitization to treatment with homeopathic remedies.

What suits your child may depend on the practical circumstances. If, for instance, your child is at a boarding school, it may not be possible for him to have a diet which avoids all wheat or dairy products. In this case, homeopathic desensitization could help (see section on Food Remedies, p.70). A course of treatment will generally run for four weeks. In the first week your child will take up to 10 drops of a specially prepared tincture three times a day. In the second week he will take a different tincture, and so on.

After desensitization, your child may try (for instance) a drink of milk – and find he no longer has any allergic or intolerance symptoms. If symptoms persist, however, you may need to take him back to the homeopath for a different course of desensitization.

Some homeopaths will also treat your child at the same time with a deep-acting remedy. This may work on deeper symptoms. For instance, the remedy you may be given for asthma may also work at a psychological level; or, it may work on internal organs, such as the bowel; it may be a constitutional remedy (i.e. one which matches the individual's symptoms of good health).

Many homeopaths will have training in other complementary disciplines and so you may also be offered one of a range of nutritional remedies (such as acidophilus if your child has been prescribed antibiotics) and/or herbal remedies (such as echinacea to lessen the toxic load on your child's body) which will work hand-in-hand with homeopathic treatment.

■ NATUROPATHY

This therapy originated in the nineteenth century and is based on maximizing the healing properties of nature. It involves nutritional advice, water therapy (or hydrotherapy, such as immersion in salt water Sitz baths), detoxification therapy, relaxation and stress management, osteopathy and cranial osteopathy, and sometimes colonic cleansing (although this is not suitable for children). Some naturopaths also incorporate homeopathy and/or herbs into their therapy. Modern naturopathy seeks to treat and avert disease by bolstering the body's defence system, primarily through a healthy diet and sensible lifestyle.

What to expect at a consultation

The practitioner will want to know all about your child. Standard medical techniques, including X-rays, blood tests and urine tests may also be used in diagnosis, and some naturopaths make an iris (of the eye) analysis (iridology).

Once a diagnosis is made, you will be advised on diet, exercise and any other treatment for your child. If a food allergy is suspected, she may have to give up whatever is causing the allergy for some time. Naturopaths regard a healthy diet – based on raw, organic food – as the best form of medicine, but this is often combined with other treatments to stimulate the body's vital force, rather than to suppress symptoms. Raw fruits and vegetables in juice form are also often prescribed.

When dealing with allergies, naturopaths may assess your child for Leaky Gut Syndrome and prescribe remedies to alleviate it.

EASTERN MEDICINE

Eastern philosophies, such as those from India, China and Tibet, believe that health is governed by energy, rather than by anatomy and physiology. Indian medicine or Ayurveda, uses the term *Prana* to describe this energy. In Traditional Chinese Medicine it is known as *Chi* which flows along 'meridians'; whereas in Tibetan medicine energy is thought to flow along 'channels'. For each system of medicine, the language is different – but the principle is much the same.

All of these systems consider hygeine, diet, exercise, breathing, meditation, manipulation (massage or manipulative techniques) and medicines to be helpful in balancing the body's energies and maintaining health.

There are more Traditional Chinese Medicine practitioners in both the UK and USA than other Eastern medicine practitioners, but methods of consultation are very similar for all kinds of Eastern medicine.

What to expect at a consultation

Diagnosis takes the form of very close observation, questioning and examination of pulses and the tongue. You will be asked about your child's lifestyle, family and health problems. His skin colour and eyes may also be inspected.

Allergic disorders such as asthma, hayfever, migraines and eczema might be treated with a detoxification programme which relates to the internal organs and body systems. Body therapies and massage may also be used.

HERBAL MEDICINE

This is often called medical or Western herbalism to distinguish it from Chinese or Ayurvedic herbalism, although they have much in common. Herbalism is one of the oldest forms of medicine and many modern drugs are based on the active elements of plants (aspirin originally comes from willow bark; morphine from poppies; digitalis from the foxglove).

Although herbalism is generally thought of as a 'gentle' therapy, herbs can have a very powerful effect, so do make sure your child takes only the preparations which have been specifically prescribed for him – and in the specific dose, no more.

If possible, your child should only take preparations which are from organically grown herbs (many commercially available herbs have been treated many times with potentially dangerous chemicals). If possible, choose a herbalist who is a trained doctor as well. See Useful Addresses.

What to expect at a consultation

Western herbalists may use several standard medical tests when making a diagnosis, as well as taking down a detailed medical history. Herbal treatments may be prescribed in the form of:

- **Tinctures** These are dried or fresh herbs steeped in water and alcohol which can be made less bitter for children by mixing with fruit juice.
- **Essential oils** These are the essential oils extracted from the plant, and bottled. These can be used in steam inhalations, in chest rubs and for massage when mixed with a carrier oil.
- **Infusions** Dried or fresh flowers and leaves are steeped in hot, freshly boiled water and left to infuse for 10 to 15 minutes. The strained tea is then drunk, one cupful three times a day.
- **Creams or compresses** These are applied topically.
- **Decoctions** This method is used to extract medicinal properties of roots, bark and twigs. These are brought to the boil in water and allowed to simmer for one hour. The strained tea is drunk, as for an infusion.

Here are a few examples of herbal remedies which are commonly used for different conditions:

For asthma

Marshmallow root can soothe and relax the airways while stimulating the immune system.
Eucalyptus oil is antiseptic and decongestant.
Chamomile is anti-inflammatory with a natural antihistamine.

For eczema

Burdock is anti-inflammatory and antibiotic.
Marigold (*Calendula officinalis*) is anti-inflammatory and strengthens the immune system.
St John's Wort (*Hypericum perforatum*) is anti-inflammatory.

For hayfever

Garlic is both antibiotic and an antihistamine.
Eyebright (*Euphrasia officinalis*) is decongestant and soothing for the mucous membranes.
Nettle (*Urticaria urens*) is anti-inflammatory when drunk as an infusion or eaten in soups.
The Chinese herb Ma Huang (*Ephedra* which contains ephedrine) is also used for a wide range of conditions.

▨ BIO-RESONANCE

As we have seen, the Eastern philosophies believe that there are energy channels or meridians throughout the body. Over the past 50 years, Western scientists have been attempting to identify this energy flow – and it seems they are getting closer to an answer.

The latest theory is that the energy which we call 'consciousness' may be created by the movement of electrons within or around micro-tubules which travel through body structures, such as nerves and bone. This theory helps to explain how bio-resonance works.

Bio-resonance machines are specialized computers which send small electric currents around your body. Certain compounds, foods and other substances can be added to the circuit of some of these machines, and their electromagnetic wavelength is then measured. In the same way, the electromagnetic impulses produced by your muscles can be measured by the computer.

Essentially, the machine's job is to measure the energy field around your child. Having done this, the computer checks his energy field against some 3,000 items to test for a reaction. These items are not all allergens – some are nutritional supplements, others are homeopathic remedies – but all help to build up a picture of your child's physical and emotional self.

The machine not only tests your child's responses, but can also treat the problems which it detects. For instance, if the computer can isolate an energy wavelength which is not normal for your child, the practitioner can use the computer to send a wavelength into your child's body which is directly opposed to the abnormal wavelength. The theory is that the two wavelengths will cancel each other out and healing results. In this way, allergies or intolerances can be switched off.

A bio-resonance machine may look quite strange to your child – rather like an electrocardiogram machine – but it is no more frightening than a computer with wires attached. Most children will happily sit still for the couple of minutes needed to do the test, with leads attached by velcro straps to the wrists and ankles. It's very unlikely that your child will feel anything; the faint pulse emitted by the machine is only 0.5 volts and while some children say they can feel it, this may be imagined.

Studies are currently in progress to assess the effectiveness of bio-resonance, but those complementary practitioners who use them say that bio-resonance machines are amazingly accurate, often revealing subtle information which patients may have withheld or forgotten to disclose. And such is the very wide range of information yielded by the machine that it takes a trained practitioner to work out exactly what to do with it.

At the very least, the machine's readout will indicate which foods and/or other substances your child should steer away from if he is to avoid allergic reactions.

While bio-resonance testing is now well established in the USA, there are still only a handful of individual complementary practitioners with access to these sophisticated computers in the UK and other parts of the Western world (see Useful Addresses).

Food remedies
According to the thinking of 'energy medicine', an allergy and/ or intolerance is the incorrect response of the body to the energy of a non-harmful substance (as opposed to the orthodox medical view that allergy is the result of the correct response of the body to harmful substances).

In energy medicine, every food substance has its own measurable energy 'resonance' which can be passed through electrical leads into a solution of water. Theoretically, the water molecule electrons pick up and retain the pattern of this resonance – and this solution becomes a remedy for allergy to the food substance. Bio-energetically prepared food remedies have yet to be subjected to scientific scrutiny, but complementary practitioners report success with them.

Food Remedies are taken under the tongue and they work on the principle of desensitization. In other words, your child's body 'recognizes' the energy resonance of the food substance, but as there is only a very small amount of resonance – and because there is no food molecule (only water) with this resonance – it learns to accept this energy as not dangerous.

ACUPUNCTURE

One of the best known and respected of complementary therapies is acupunture. It is part of a comprehensive system of Traditional Chinese Medicine which dates back thousands of years. However, in the West, acupuncture is often used on its own and many conventional health professionals have learned the techniques.

As we have seen in the section on Eastern medicine, the philosophy behind TCM and acupuncture is completely different from that of Western medical thinking. According to

Chinese beliefs, the key to health lies in the balance between two opposing forces (*Yin* and *Yang*, the passive and the active forces). Achieving balance and harmony is the fundamental objective of this complex and sophisticated system of medicine which emphasizes the close interaction of mind and body.

Healthy balance relies on the smooth flow of vital energy or *Chi* through meridians in the body. Imbalance or ill-health occurs when there are blockages or weaknesses in the flow of this energy, or if outside influences like excessive heat, cold or damp get into the body.

Acupuncture involves using very fine needles which are inserted at strategic points (acupoints) on the body to stimulate the flow of vital energy and correct imbalances.

What to expect at a consultation

Treatment is preceded by very careful questioning and observation. The practitioner will look at how your child moves, his size and so on. She will also listen very carefully not only to the anwers your child gives, but also to how your child answers – i.e. her tone and general responses. The practitioner will inspect your child's tongue and will also feel up to 14 pulses on her wrists, taking down details of her medical history, lifestyle, sleep patterns, eating habits, likes and dislikes. From this she will decide on a course of treatment.

Naturally enough, parents worry that acupuncture may hurt, but all your child should feel is a pinprick as the needles are inserted and a sensation of tingling or numbness. Initially, the needles are only left in for 6–10 minutes, building to 20–25 minutes in later sessions. Your child may feel sleepy after a session, but this is quite normal.

Acupuncture without needles
Known as 'acupuncture without needles', there are various treatments based on stimulating the acupoints which are more suitable for children who may be alarmed by the needles of traditional acupuncture.

- **Acupressure** This involves pressing on the acupoints.
- **Shiatsu** A Japanese variation of the same basic treatment, involving a clothed massage in which the practitioner pushes on the acupressure points and stretches the body's meridians.
- **Laser acupuncture** The skin does not have to be broken; instead of needles, a small pen-like instrument is simply held on the acupoint and a low-dose laser beam is used to stimulate it. The patient feels nothing. This is also becoming more widely available for children, as is:
- **Ultrasound acupuncture**.

PSYCHOLOGICAL THERAPIES

There is currently a great deal of research into the question of how the psyche affects our nervous system – which in turn controls our immune system by affecting the thymus, pituitary and adrenal glands. (This field is known as psycho-neuro-immunology or PNI.)

As parents we are aware of how the stresses of daily life can affect our children's psyches. Problems such as bullying, being slow at school, being 'unsporting', dyslexic – or simply different – do put tremendous pressure on children. We may be less aware of how 'an ordinary argument' (in adult terms) can cause children a great deal of stress – especially when the argument is between their mother and father.

Stress causes the release of two hormones: adrenaline and cortisol. Adrenaline speeds up the body, uses up nutrients and can lead to deficiencies in vitamin B_6 (pyridoxine), amino acids, zinc and tryptophan (deficiencies of which are implicated in depression). All of these changes can lead to a weakening of the immune system.

Cortisol, known as the body's 'natural steroid', is an immune suppressant. You might think that suppressing the immune response would be no bad thing when dealing with allergies or intolerances, but unfortunately, when cortisol diminishes, the body goes into 'rebound', creating an even stronger inflammatory response – the last thing an allergic child needs.

Psychological techniques which reduce stress in a child's life can therefore be very effective in combating allergies. The best of these are known as 'counselling with an angle' and they include art, music, dance and drama therapy. These are particularly suitable for children because they involve fun and play.

Another psychological technique which can help children with allergies is hypnotherapy. This is a technique involving deep relaxation which enables the subconscious part of the mind to express itself and to receive messages in order to bring about change. It is used to treat a wide range of stress-related disorders – including allergies and intolerances – in children over the age of five years.

If your child is suffering from the kind of stress which follows discord in the family, couples counselling can be very useful, not only to help you resolve relationship problems, but also to help you become aware of how conflict at home may be affecting your child.

BREATHING TECHNIQUES

For five thousand years, Eastern philosophies of health have regarded breathing as absolutely central to staying well. This section looks at three breathing techniques which can help children with allergies; the best known of these is yoga.

Remedial Yoga

As usually practised in the West, yoga aims to bring the body back to a more centred and balanced response to our environment. Yoga breathing – amongst other things – has the healing effect of moving blocked *Chi* (energy). Yoga can also be valuable in treating allergies because it helps to reduce the effects of stress which, as we have seen, can have damaging effects on health. Yoga is generally seen as an adult leisure pursuit in the West, although it can be very appealing to children: many of the yoga postures, for instance, are fun to do and are named after animals.

Oxygenesis

This is a technique in which individuals learn (over 6 to 10 sessions) the ideal breathing pattern for themselves. It is based on the fact that some of us breathe too frequently; others too deeply. This easy-to-learn technique has been developed in California and is very new in the UK, but in the future it may prove to be of benefit for many conditions (see Useful Addresses).

The Buteyko Method

This is based on the theory that many illnesses – including asthma and allergies – are caused by 'overbreathing'. It was developed by a Russian medical scientist, Dr Konstantin Butyeko, some 40 years ago when he observed that patients with breathing disorders and allergies all breathed more than normal. He concluded that deep breathing was not just a symptom but a cause of their ailments. The technique he developed is a series of exercises designed to restore breathing patterns to a normal level by retraining the body's involuntary respiratory centre in the brain.

Low carbon dioxide levels have a direct effect on the immune system because it is one of the key regulatory chemicals in the body. The Buteyko theory is that a deficiency of carbon dioxide means that the body's antigens do not bind to foreign material as fast as they should. In some allergies, the body has become super-sensitive to a given substance. Correcting the carbon dioxide levels can bring the threshold of sensitivity back to normal.

Buteyko treatment involves one-hour sessions, usually in a workshop (although one-to-one sessions are available) for five consecutive days. It begins with a simple 'control pause' test, to see how long your child can comfortably hold his breath. It moves on to a series of breath-holding exercises which must be practised to maintain good health. This therapy is very popular in Australia, although it is still not widely available in the UK or USA.

Buteyko practitioners claim it can dramatically 'cure' asthma and allergies within the space of a week, while many of their colleagues in complementary medicine are watching the ongoing studies into the method with interest.

SUPPORTING THERAPIES

Aromatherapy and massage

Aromatic essential oils extracted from parts of plants or trees have been used for thousands of years for healing and promoting a general feeling of relaxation and well being.

Essential oils are often used in massage, a manipulation therapy which can balance and relax the whole of the body, helping alleviate the symptoms of allergy. For example:

• Peppermint is often used to relieve hayfever symptoms

(although it cannot be used in conjunction with homeopathy)

- Chamomile and lemon balm are useful both for hayfever and for allergic skin reactions.
- Frankincense is used for both hayfever and asthma.
- Neroli can be used in the bath to relieve eczema.
- Lavender promotes relaxation; use it in the bath or put a few drops on your child's pillow to help him to sleep.
- Geranium in the bath can be used to combat eczema.

Flower remedies

Flower essences have a vibrational energy which helps to guard against sickness and disease by balancing the (negative) emotions that cause or aggravate so many chronic disorders and prevent the body from healing. A trained therapist will select an appropriate mix of remedies that will correspond to your child's particular emotions and condition. For example:

- Crab apple may be suggested if your child suffers from dermatitis and feels self-conscious about his appearance.
- Green rose or Lantana are often used for hayfever.
- Eucalyptus is used for asthma, together with Grape Hyacinth and Babies' breath.
- Luffa is used to cleanse the system and to combat eczema.

Healing

Healing works on the assumption that the electromagnetic energy of a patient can be altered by those of us with a specific healing power. The healer acts as a channel for what they consider a higher source of energy and transfers it – often via his or her hands – to the patient, rebalancing the particular frequencies which are generated by the individuals' internal organs. As energy involves heat, patients often report a warm tingling sensation as well as feelings of calm and relaxation.

Scientific research has found that during the healing process, the healer's brainwave frequency – and then the patient's – change to 'alpha', a state of relaxed awareness comparable to that found during meditation. You may feel better immediately after healing, or it could be days before you feel any effect.

Chapter Six

As They Grow

As we have seen, there are many ways in which you can help your allergic child, but your child's needs – and your response – will vary as she grows from baby to toddler to child to teenager. For instance, it will be your responsibility for many years to make sure she takes any necessary medication, but as she grows up you will need to hand over the responsibility gradually to her.

There will be important stages in your child's life too, heralding major changes which may well affect her allergies and the way you handle them. As your child starts school for instance, she will learn to cope with her condition in a new environment. As she becomes a teenager and then a young adult, encountering new friends and relationships, going through the stresses of examinations and job interviews, you will have a whole new range of challenges to face.

Remember, too, that many of the common allergies and intolerances – including asthma, eczema and hayfever – will come and go depending on your child's age. As the years pass, symptoms often lessen or disappear altogether. Some 30 per cent of children with asthma, for instance, find during their teens that they are 'in remission' (as opposed to 'cured' – because the symptoms may return later in life). Another third will find that their symptoms lessen, or that they have fewer asthma attacks.

As the years go by you may also find a complementary therapy which suits your child and puts and end to allergy and intolerance once and for all.

Apart from the relief of knowing that allergies and/or intolerances need not be a 'life sentence', this means that the strategies parents devise for dealing with allergies will change as their children grow. This Chapter outlines some of those changes and suggests ways that you can stay on top of the situation – until your child is a child no longer.

■ PRECONCEPTUAL CARE AND PREGNANCY

Increasingly, medical specialists are recognizing that the months before conception – as well as the nine months of pregnancy – can be crucial in determining the future health of your child. If you have allergies and/or intolerances in the family already, it is all the more important to take steps to protect your baby – and there are many practical measures you can take.

We know that allergies/intolerances run in families, but what your child inherits is only a *tendency* to allergy. Whether she develops a full-blown allergy or not depends very much on her diet and environment not only in the sensitive weeks and months after birth, but also while still in the womb.

Case Study
Why does my child have an allergy to nuts?

Sally's son Jason has a severe nut allergy, and like many parents, Sally has often wondered about the reasons:

'Allergies don't run in my family or my husband's, so I wondered *why*? It could be that he was sensitized while in my womb; I ate a lot of brazil nuts when I was pregnant and I also cooked a lot of nut roasts. I'm told there is often peanut products in commercial baby food – as well as in some of the preparations which I used to alleviate nipple soreness when I was breastfeeding.'

The allergic reaction that many parents are most anxious to avoid is anaphylactic shock (see p.46). This potentially deadly and increasingly common reaction is often the result of eating peanuts or peanut products. An estimated one person in 200 in the UK alone is now allergic to peanuts, causing a number of dramatic deaths each year.

The latest medical advice is directed at preventing peanut allergy from developing in the first place:

- Pregnant women should avoid eating peanuts or peanut containing foods if they, their partners or a previous child suffers from a diagnosed allergy such as asthma, eczema or hay fever.
- Breastfeeding mothers are also sometimes advised not to eat any peanut containing foods.
- Children with a family history of allergic conditions are also being advised to avoid peanuts until they are about three years old.
- If you are breastfeeding, it is also worth avoiding the nipple creams and other skin creams that contain peanut oil – likely to be described as 'arachis oil' on the label. It seems likely that newborns – who are very easily sensitized to allergens absorbed even in small amounts – could develop peanut allergy in this way.
- Many of the commercial creams made for infants – including those for eczema, nappy rash and cradle cap – may also contain peanut oil, so do ask your doctor or pharmacist for an alternative.

▨ THE PRE-SCHOOL YEARS: FROM BIRTH TO FIVE

▨ The First Year

At birth, your baby's immune system is still immature and your breastmilk contains the antibodies she needs to fight off bacteria and viruses. But to let these antibodies through into her blood-stream your baby's gut is 'leaky' or permeable. Not only the antibodies from breastmilk can get through the gut, however, but all sorts of food particles which have not been fully digested can get into your baby's blood through her gut as well.

This means that any form of food taken in by your baby in the first three months is absorbed into her bloodstream. If she is bottle-fed, or if you give her 'solids' at a very early age, the proteins in the milk formula (usually based on cow's milk) and other foods will go into her immature system – and may cause an allergic reaction.

The best advice, especially if allergies and/or intolerances run in your family, is to:

- **Breastfeed your baby** for at least six months, longer if possible, and give your baby nothing but breastmilk for the first four to six months. Breastfeeding not only nurtures a close emotional bond between you and your baby, it provides the best possible form of nutrition and protection against all sorts of illnesses and infections – including allergy. Scientists have never been able to replicate the many subtle properties of breastmilk which include protective antibodies and just the right balance of nutrients, varying as your baby grows, to help her develop in the best possible health.

  As we have seen, if you have food allergies and/or intolerances in your family, avoid the common allergy-causing foods while you are breastfeeding, as whatever you eat or drink finds its way into breastmilk.

  If you do have problems getting breastfeeding started – or keeping going – don't lose heart. You can get support and advice from a network of organizations including the

National Childbirth Trust in the UK (see Useful Addresses) who have many locally based breastfeeding counsellors, and the La Leche League in the UK, USA, Australia and Canada.

- **Introduce solids slowly,** in small quantities and one at a time – while still breastfeeding. Parents often feel pressured to get their babies onto solid food, but it is not a race. Remember that breastmilk is a complete food which automatically adjusts itself to your baby's needs, depending on her age and stage of development – an extraordinary advantage which no babyfood manufacturer can ever match.

  When you do start weaning, offer only very bland foods like baby rice and (whenever possible) home-cooked and organic puréed apples and pears. Avoid the common allergy-causing foods and all glutens (including cereals and biscuits) until *at least six months*. The foods most likely to cause a problem for small children and babies are unfortunately the ones they often come across first.

  The Health Education Authority (UK) advises parents to avoid giving the following foods to babies until they are *at least six months old*. A working party set up by the World Health Authority recommends that children should avoid these foods until they are one year old:
- Wheat
- Rye
- Barley
- Fish
- Soya
- Citrus fruits
- Nuts and sesame seeds
- Beef and chicken may also cause problems.
- **Avoid cow's milk products until your child is one year old.** Cow's milk is so often associated with allergic reactions that if allergies run in your family, it is best to carry on with either breastmilk or soya formula milk, slowly increasing the amount of solids, until your child is at least one. Try using expressed breastmilk to mix with cereals, mashed potato and other foods.

Case Study
Jo's four-year-old son Ricky has eczema, occasional asthma attacks, and reacts badly to certain foods:

'We keep him off all dairy products because of his eczema, and we avoid sugary foods too. But when he goes to friends' houses and eats sweets you can see the change in his behaviour. He comes home wide-eyed and twitching. He can't settle to anything and we just have to give him space to run it off. We've talked about it with him and we call it "busy brain". But it is hard to restrict children entirely; you want mealtimes and food to be happy times.'

The Pre-School Years

Food can be a major battleground in any family – allergic/ intolerant or not – with parents coaxing toddlers to sit still long enough to eat up and older sibling taking full advantage of their parents' anxieties to get as much attention as possible. Add a food allergy or intolerance into the fray and you've got a potent emotional mix with important health and nutritional implications. Children of two or three or even four years are very unlikely to accept with good grace that their sibling can have a fruit yogurt/piece of cake/ helping of ice cream – but that they can't for the good of their health.

There is no easy answer to the dilemmas of family mealtimes with an allergic and/or intolerant child. One alternative, though, that you might like to consider is that the whole family eats the same food so that no one feels left out. But as ever with small children, if you can stay calm and be consistently firm, life will be easier in the long run. You may well have to face out a few tantrums and refusals of meals, but remember that no child deliberately starves herself for long. Remember, too, that no matter how upset your child may become, when it comes to her health and her diet, you really do know best. If you feel that, despite your best efforts, she is missing out on important nutrients, you could supplement her diet with the appropriate vitamin and minerals in tablet or syrup form.

And if you feel thoroughly fed-up with always having to say

'No', why not try a more creative approach. If your child can't eat cakes with eggs in them, find a recipe for eggless cakes – and ask your child to help you cook the 'special recipe'. The trick is to make her feel special – and deserving of special food – not that she is missing out.

The same holds true, of course, for other allergens. Perhaps she is allergic to cats and so can't have any pets at home – but if she doesn't react to horses, then regular riding lessons would be a great bonus. If playing in the garden becomes a problem during peak hayfever season, pick a special family holiday by the sea or in the hills where pollen counts are lower. An allergy to house dust mites may mean no curtains in her bedroom, but she could have some truly fashionable blinds instead!

Hyperactivity

One aspect of allergy and intolerance which causes parents a great deal of anxiety is that of so-called hyperactivity – not least because it is so difficult to pin down. Children who are hyperactive are typically overactive and excitable, constantly fidgeting and easily distracted. They may also be irritable, and prone to temper tantrums, sleep poorly and sometimes become agressive and destructive. Hyperactivity is also known as hyperkinetic syndrome; ADD or Attention Deficit Disorder; and as ADHD or Attention Deficit and Hyperactivity Disorder.

The trouble is that *all* small children show aspects of this kind of behaviour at some time or another, depending on whether they are feeling stressed, frustrated or simply tired. The trick is to establish the difference between behaviour which is within the 'normal' range, and that which is persistent enough to indicate a problem. It may be, of course, that your child is simply very bright with a vivid imagination but frustrated in her attempts at expressing herself, with the result that she appears over-energetic and even out of control. An absorbing constructive task (perhaps with a grandparent) can work wonders. Often the problem resolves once the child starts school. However, if you suspect that there *is* a problem, try to monitor the behaviour. One way of doing this is to keep a diary, noting what your child eats, where she has been/what she has been doing – and how she is behaving. If you suspect that certain foods and/or drinks are the cause, an elimination diet can bring dramatic improvement within a few weeks. There is evidence that enzyme potentiated desensitization (EPD) may also help (see p.50.)

Case Study

As a baby, Lynn's son Sam rarely slept for more than an hour or two at a stretch. As he grew into a hyperactive toddler, she began to suspect that his diet was at the root of the problem:

'When he was a toddler he used to have so much excess energy that he literally used to run into walls, bang! He'd fall down, get up, turn around – and run into another one. It was a nightmare: I could never leave him with anyone else and his younger sister was often ignored as we tried to deal with Sam. By watching him very carefully, I worked out that it was dairy products which set him off. When I cut them out of his diet for a few weeks at a stretch he was so much better.

As he has grown older we have identified, by trial and error, other sensitivities. When he goes to friends' houses and has sweets or fizzy drinks many of the symptoms come back. He gets home and can't relax or sleep. We've identified sodium benzoate, which is in many fizzy drinks, as one of his triggers. I've also realized that I was allergic as a child. I remember always having this whirring feeling inside; it must have been adrenaline. As an adult I used to get a lot of migraines and headaches, but they are much better since I have cut out dairy products too.'

Childcare

Parents of children with allergies and/or intolerances have to make not only the usual choices about what is best for their child, but other important decisions, too, such as what to do about using a childminder or enrolling her in a playgroup or preschool nursery.

The most important step is to talk to your chid's carer (or playgroup leader or teacher) about how she is going to deal with any problems caused by your child's allergy. Provide important health information – such as details about medication – in writing. Keep the lines of communication open: a few minutes' chat a couple of times a week can make all the difference.

Checklist for childcare

When your child starts nursery or goes to a childminder, make sure that your child's carer:

- Knows what to do if your child has an allergic reaction such as an asthma attack. This is especially important if there is any risk of anaphylaxsis.
- Is willing and able to give medication on a regular basis if necessary, or is willing to administer emergency medication for anaphylaxis such as an adrenaline (epinephrine) injection.
- Can adapt the environment of home or nursery to make sure there are no potential allergens such as pet dander, or cigarette smoke.

You will also need to consider whether certain activities may make her condition worse – and whether you are prepared to take that risk. If she has eczema for instance, playing with sand and water may be bad for her skin. The kind of modelling materials used at playgroups may also set off a reaction. If she is allergic to furry animals, visits to your local farm or animal centre may also trigger her allergy.

Small children love baking and many playgroups and

childminders spend a lot of time making biscuits and cakes with children. Let your child's carers know if your child reacts badly to eggs (for instance), and suggest alternative recipes.

However, small children do need – and want – to take part in most of the normal activities of childhood. Getting whole-heartedly involved in fun and shared activities not only helps distract your child from her symptoms, it is often more 'healthy' than dwelling on the problems of allergy.

THE MIDDLE YEARS: FROM FIVE TO TWELVE

Starting school

As we have heard from many children in this book, having an allergy and/or intolerance is considered to be quite common by today's youngsters who know many others at school with similar difficulties. Unfortunately, many schools don't seem to have quite caught up with the rise in children's allergies and intoler-ances and their attitude to your child's health – and especially medication – may seem unsupportive if not antagonistic.

Few schools have a policy on dealing with allergic reactions, such as asthma, and surveys show that many teachers have little understanding of the condition. This makes it all the more important that you should communicate early, often and clearly with your child's school. Be especially clear about any form of medication your child requires – especially if there is any risk of anaphylaxsis.

Food is going to be an issue at school, too. Parents of children with food allergies and intolerances may need to prepare suitable packed lunches – and make sure that teachers and/or carers are aware of the potential dangers of the allergy. This is especially important if your child has a severe allergy to nuts. Lunchboxes may not be a hardship, however; with a little originality and imagination you can get together a package which will be the envy of your child's burger-and-chips-eating friends!

Sport, games and extracurricular activities are an important part of children's school lives, not only in terms of having fun and developing friendships, but to keep them healthy and strong too. A good level of general fitness can help your child to stay robust, enjoy life and fight off any infections that may come her way.

A good social life can also be very stimulating. Within a short time, it is likely that friends will start asking your child home to play after school. This means that she will be exposed to various allergens – such as pets, dust mites and certain foods – which may cause a reaction. You may worry about the consequences, but rather than preventing your child from joining in with her peers, try to ensure that she knows what foods or substances will trigger her allergy, so that she can steer clear of them. If she feels shy about making this clear to friends' parents, you could coach her in what she should say – and you could also give the parents a ring to reinforce the message!

These years are crucial in helping your child to develop a positive, confident self-image and any suggestion by the staff in a school that she is 'not normal' can be very damaging and will need to be challenged. Make sure that your child's school is not preventing her from joining in any activities because of her allergies/intolerances, and that she is not being made conspicuous by constantly having to ask her teacher/the school nurse for her asthma inhaler, for instance.

Some teachers may harbour prejudicial and/or inaccurate attitudes towards intolerances or allergic reactions such as asthma, suggesting that symptoms are 'all in the mind' or 'put on'. If your child encounters attitudes like this, don't ignore what has happened. Speak to the teacher or headteacher, challenge these ideas and set the record straight. Children with allergy or intolerance deserve sensitivity and understanding from their teachers at the very least.

> **School and medical emergencies**
> Different schools may have very different policies on how to deal with severe allergic reactions. Jason, who has a potentially fatal allergy to nuts, has moved from one primary school to another, and his mother has had detailed discussions with teacher at both:
> 'They have been very good at his current primary school. We went in to talk to the staff about his allergic reactions and we also arranged for an allergy specialist to go into the school to discuss it with them. One of the members of staff is now trained and ready to deal with an emergency; she is able to administer the EpiPen (a measured dose of adrenaline by injection), which is very reassuring for us.
> At our previous primary school they didn't want to deal with an emergency themselves, but they did advise three local health centres to be on standby in case he needed help.'

THE TEENAGE YEARS FROM 13–18

Many parents of teenagers will tell you that this is a rollercoaster time for the whole family – whether your child has any health problems or not! Not only are young people struggling with changes in their bodies, they are often also extremely volatile emotionally. Adolescence is a time when your children can't yet cope with the outside world without you, yet most of the time would rather die than be seen in your company! This, not surprisingly, causes family tensions – and when potential allergic reactions are also involved, it can be an explosive mixture!

Janet's daughter Kelly has severe allergies including asthma. 'The difficulty with teenagers is to get them to stick to their treatment programme,' she says. 'Kelly does try to be very positive, but she goes through phases where she just can't be bothered.'

Ann's son Gareth had severe food allergies as a child: 'You know how they are as teenagers,' says Ann. 'There's no telling him what to do and I find the best policy is to say nothing but to keep an eye on him. He goes off to friends' houses and eats things that he shouldn't; I always know because he gets over-emotional. But he is learning from experience and most of the time now he sticks to a sensible diet.'

There are positive sides to the changes of adolescence, too – increased independence, for example, and personal achievements. As Janet has discovered: 'We try to be very positive too and we encourage her interest in swimming – she got her gold recently – and her flute playing, which has helped her breathing no end. And she climbed to the top of Snowdon recently with her Venture group, not by the easy route either!'

There is good news about puberty too; because, for many, this is a time when their allergic and/or intolerance symptoms fade or become easier to manage. For others, symptoms disappear never to return.

Leaving home

Increased independence can seem like a mixed blessing to parents who have watched so carefully over their child's health for many years. Indeed, it can be hard to let go. As Jason's mother puts it:

'He still gets fed up at parties when he can't eat the same food as the others, but he is very good about it. The other day we went on a picnic and his father had bought some Easter biscuits without checking them for nuts. Jason said, "Oh, I won't have any then." '

'We've got a special allergy pack for him that his doctor put together. It contains an EpiPen, plus extra phials of adrenaline (epinephrine) and syringes – everything he would need in the event of an attack together with instructions on how to use them. But I do worry that when he gets older and leaves home he may go out drinking with his mates, go with them for an Indian meal – forgetting that many curries have nuts or nut products in them – and have a severe reaction. His allergy comes on very quickly and it is very serious. But for the time being I think we have done all that we can to keep him safe.'

Kelly's mother has similar feelings:

'In a few years she'll be going away to college and I won't be there to run around after her checking that she's got her medicines, so she has to learn to stand on her own two feet. I do worry an awful lot about her [she also has a severe peanut allergy], but as she's getting older I am letting her take more control. I've got to hand over the responsibility to her. Even six months ago I was reminding her – "Have you taken this or that treatment," but not any more. Although it is difficult, I have to let her go.'

For young people with allergies, leaving home means finally taking full responsibility for their health. It is a big step, and you will not be there to check that they get it right. But they will have learned from your attitude that they can take control of their allergies and intolerances, can look after themselves, stay well, and enjoy life to the full. With confidence and a positive approach, your child is set to make the most of life's opportunities and you have done your very best in preparing her to take her place in the world.

Conclusion

As we have seen in this book, when it comes to allergy and intolerance, there is a very wide range of treatments – both conventional and complementary – to choose from. If you have a sympathetic family doctor, you may be fortunate enough to identify the problem – and hit on the right kind of medication to relieve your child's symptoms – at an early stage. If your search takes you into the realms of complementary medicine, you may also gain insight into the deeper causes of your child's condition, and (as happens in some cases) you may even discover a cure.

Whatever course of action you decide to take, becoming well informed on the subject will enable you to ask the right questions of your doctor and/or complementary practitioner, as well as helping you to feel less stressed and more in control of the situation. And the more in control you feel, the more you will be able to help your child. A more relaxed you means a more relaxed child, with positive health benefits for all the family! An added bonus of many of the complementary treatments for allergy and intolerance is that they can involve making positive changes in your lifestyles – especially diet – which can make your whole family healthier in the long run.

Last but not least, the very fact that you have taken the trouble to find out all you can about the possible causes and treatments of your child's condition will bring you closer. Of course there will be problems along the way, but time is on your side and meanwhile, your care and attention to the subject is healing in itself!

Appendix

Food groups

Apple Apple, pear, quince, loquat, pectin, cider.

Amaranthaceae Amaranth.

Arum Dasheen, eddoes.

Aster Lettuce, chicory, endive, globe and Jerusalem artichoke, dandelion, sunflower, salsify, tarragon, curry leaves, camomile, yarrow, safflower oil.

Banana Banana, plantain, arrowroot.

Beech Chestnuts.

Beef Beef, veal, all cows' milk products. Lamb/mutton, goat and milk products.

Beet Sugar beet, spinach, Swiss chard, beetroot.

Birch Filberts, hazelnuts, birch oil (wintergreen).

Bird All fowl and game birds, including chicken, turkey, duck, goose, pigeon, quail, pheasant, partridge, grouse, eggs.

Blueberry Blueberry, cranberry.

Buckwheat Buckwheat, rhubarb, sorrel, amaranth (nearest family).

Caper Caper.

Cashew Cashew, pistachio, mango.

Citrus Lemon, orange, grapefruit, lime, tangerine, citron.

Conifer Juniper, pine nuts.

Crustacean Crab, crayfish, lobster, prawn, shrimp.

Cyperacea Tiger nuts.

Deer Venison.
Dillenia Kiwi fruit (Chinese gooseberry).
Elderberry Elderberry.
Flax Linseed (flax).
Freshwater fish Salmon, trout, pike, perch, bass.
Fungus Mushrooms, yeast.
Ginger East Indian arrowroot, ginger, cardamom, turmeric.
Gooseberry Currant, gooseberry.
Grape Grapes, raisins, sultanas, wine, (cream of tartar).
Grass Wheat, spelt wheat, corn (maize), oats, barley, rye, rice, malt, millet, quinoa, bamboo shoots, sugar cane, sorghum, kamut.
Laurel Avocado, cinnamon, bay leaves.
Lily Onion, garlic, asparagus, chives, leeks.
Madder Coffee.
Mallow Okra, hibiscus.
Maple Maple syrup.
Melon Watermelon, cantaloupe and other melons, cucumber, zucchini, marrow, pumpkin, acorn squash and other squashes.
Mint Apple mint, basil, bergamot, hyssop, lavender, lemon balm, marjoram, oregano, peppermint, rosemary, sage, spearmint, savory, thyme.
Mollusc Abalone, snail, squid, clam, mussel, oyster, scallop, octopus.
Morning glory Sweet potato.
Mulberry Figs, mulberry, hops, breadfruit.
Mustard Turnip, swede, radish, daikon, horseradish, Chinese leaves, watercress, mustard and cress, cabbage, cauliflower, broccoli, Brussels sprouts, kohlrabi, kale, mustard seed, rape seed.
Myrtle Allspice, cloves, guava.
Nutmeg Nutmeg, mace.
Olive Black or green olives.
Orchid Vanilla.

Palm Coconut, date, date sugar, sago.

Papaya Papaya.

Parsley Carrots, parsnips, celery, celeriac, fennel, anise, parsley, caraway, lovage, chervil, coriander, cumin, dill.

Pea Pea, sugar peas, mangetout, runner beans, French beans, broad beans, dried beans (*aduki beans, black beans, black-eyed beans, butter beans, cannellini beans, chickpeas, flageolet beans, haricot beans, lima beans, mung beans, dried peas, split green peas, split yellow peas, pinto beans, red kidney beans, soya beans*), lentils (*brown lentils, continental lentils, puy lentils, split red lentils*), alfalfa sprouts, liquorice, peanuts, fenugreek, red clover, senna, carob, Rooibosch tea.

Pedalium Sesame seeds.

Pepper Black and white pepper, peppercorn.

Pineapple Pineapple.

Plum Plum, damson, sloe, cherry, peach, apricot, nectarine, prune, almond.

Potato Potato, tomato, aubergine (eggplant), peppers (capsicum), paprika, cayenne, chilli, tobacco.

Protea Macadamia nuts.

Rabbit Hare, rabbit.

Rose Strawberry, raspberry, blackberry, loganberry, rosehip.

Saltwater fish Tuna, mackerel, herring, eel, halibut, turbot, anchovy, sardine and pilchard, whitebait, sprats, sea bass, plaice, sole, cod, hake, haddock, sea bream, mullet.

Seaweed Arame, nori, carrageen, wakeman, dulse, kelp, kombu, agar-agar.

Soapberry Lychees.

Spurge Cassava (tapioca).

Sterculia Cocoa.

Subucaya Brazil nut.

Swine Pork, wild boar.

Tea Tea, green leaf tea.

Walnut Walnut, hickory nut, butternut, pecan.

Water chestnut Water chestnut.
Yam Yam.
Verbenum Lemon verbena.

Reprinted with the permission of Jill Carter and Alison Edwards from The Elimination Diet Cookbook (1997).

Further Reading

The Complete Guide to Food Allergy and Intolerance by Professor Jonathon Brostoff and Linda Gamlin (Bloomsbury, 1989)

The Element Family Encyclopedia of Health by Dr Rajendra Sharma (Element, 1998)

The Elimination Diet Cook Book by Jill Carter and Alison Edwards (Element, 1997)

HEA Guide to Complementary Medicines and Therapies by Anne Woodham (HEA, 1994)

Natural Remedies for Allergies by Paul Morgan (Parragon, 1995)

The Rotation Diet Cookbook by Jill Carter and Alison Edwards (Element, 1997)

Useful Addresses

Australia

Allergy Association Australia
PO Box 214
North Beach
WA 6020

Allergy Recognition and Management
PO Box 2
Sandy Bay
Tasmania 7005

Australian Natural Therapists Association
7 Highview Grove
Burwood East
VIC 3151

Australian Traditional Medicine Society
120 Blaxland Road
Ryde
NSW 2112

Marriage and Family Counselling Service
2262 Pitt Street
Sydney
NSW 2000

Nursing Mothers Association of Australia
16 Dinsdale Place
Hamersley
WA 6022

Canada

AIA Allergy Information Association
3 Powburn Place
Weston
Ontario

Canadian Holistic Medical Association
42 Redpath Avenue
Toronto
Ontario
M4S 2J6

Secrétariat Général de la Léche League
CF P 874
Ville St Laurent
Quebec
H4L 4WS

Canadian Institute of Stress
1235 Bay Street
Toronto
Ontario
M5R 3K4

Ireland

Irish Allergy Association
PO Box 1067
Churchtown
Dublin

New Zealand

Allergy Awareness Association
PO Box 120701
Penrose
Auckland 6

New Zealand Natural Health Practitioners Accreditation Board
PO Box 37–491
Auckland
Tel: 9 625 9966
Supported by 15 therapy organizations

United Kingdom

Dr R Sharma and The 101 Practitioners Network
87 North Road
Parkstone
Poole
Dorset
BH14 0LT
Tel: 01425 461 740
Network of complementary practitioners trained and experienced in many of the therapies outlined in Chapter 5.

Action Against Allergy
43 The Downs
London
SW20

Anaphlaxis Campaign
PO Box 149
Fleet
Hampshire
GU13 9XU

Aromatherapy Organisations Council
3 Latymer Close
Braybrooke
Market Harborough
Leics
LE16 8LN
Tel: 01858 434242

Biolab Medical Diagnostic Laboratory
Stone House
9 Weymouth Street
London W1N 3FF
Gut permeability test for Leaky Gut Syndrome

British Acupuncture Council
Park House
206/208 Latimer Road
London
W10 6RE
Tel: 0181 964 0222

British Allergy Foundation
Tel: 0181 303 8525

British Association for Counselling
37a Sheep Street
Rugby
Warks
CV21 3BX
Tel: 01788 578328

British Digestive Foundation
3 St Andrew's Place
London
NW1 4LB
Tel: 0171 487 5332

British Homoeopathic Association
27a Devonshire Street
London
W1N 3FF
Tel: 0171 935 2163
Medically qualified homeopaths only

British Massage Therapy Council
Greenbank House
65a Adelphi St
Preston
PR1 7BH
Tel: 01772 881063

British Wheel of Yoga
1 Hamilton Place
Boston Road
Sleaford
Lincs
NG34 7ES
Tel: 01529 306851

British Society for Allergy, Environment and Nutritional Medicine
Tel: 01703 812124

British Society for Nutritional Medicine
Stone House
9 Weymouth Street
London
W1N 3FF
Tel: 0171 436 8532

General Council and Register of Consultant Herbalists
18 Sussex Square
Brighton
East Sussex
BN2 5AA

Individual Well-being Diagnostic Laborative
1 Cadogan Gardens
London
SW3 2RJ
Tel: 0171 730 7010
(10% discount on the FACT tests if you quote this book).

Institute for Complementary Medicine
PO Box 194
London
SE14 1QZ
Tel: 0171 237 5165

The Institute for Optimum Nutrition
Blades Court
Deodar Road
London
SW15 2NU

The Institute of Stress Management
57 Hall Lane
London
NW4 4TJ
Tel: 0171 203 7355

La Leche League
BM 3424
London
WC1V 6XX
Tel: 0171 242 1278
Support for breastfeeding mothers

National Asthma Campaign
Providence House
Providence Place
London
N1 0NT
Asthma helpline: 0345 010203
Tel: 0171 226 2269

National Asthma Training Centre
Winton House
Church Street
Stratford-upon-Avon
Warwickshire
CV37 6HB

National Council of Psychotherapists and Hypnotherapists
46 Oxhey Road
Oxhey,
Watford
Herts
WD1 4QQ

National Eczema Society
163 Eversholt Street
London
NW1 1BU
Tel: 0171 978 6278

National Institute of Medical Herbalism
Tel: 0113 924 26022

Osteopathic Information Service
PO Box 2074
Reading
Berks
RG1 4YR
Tel: 01491 875255

Society for the Promotion of Nutritional Therapy (SPNT)
PO Box 47
Heathfield
East Sussex
TN21 8ZX

USA

Allergy Foundation of America
801 Second Avenue
New York
NY 10017

American Association of Naturopathic Physicians
2800 East Madison Street
Suite 200
Seattle
Washington 98112
or
PO Box 20386
Seattle
Washington 98102
Tel: 206 323 7610
Fax: 206 323 7612

International Academy of Environmental Medicine
Prairie Village
Kansas
Tel: 913 642 6062

Internal Academy of Nutrition and Preventative Medicine
PO Box 5832
Lincoln
Nebraska 68505
Tel: 402 467 2716

La Leche League International
PO Box 1209
Franklin Park
IL 601310–8209

National Anxiety Foundation
3135 Custer Drive
Lexington
Kentucky 40517

—

Index

Note: where more than one reference is given, main references are indicated in **bold**.

acidophilus 19, 64
acupressure 72
acupuncture 61, **70–2**
additives 4
adolescence 90–2
adrenaline (epinephrine) 38, 43–4, 50, 72
Aerolin 43
ALCAT (Antigen, Leucocyte Cellular Antibody Test) 40
alcohol 34
allergic reactions 1–2
allergy tests 39–41, 57–9
Anapen 50
anaphylaxis 31, 37–8, **49–50**, 81
animal allergens 22, 85
antibiotics 19, 47
antibodies 2
antigens 1
antihistamines 47, 48, 50
arachis oil 81
aromatherapy 35, 61, **75–6**
art therapy 73
asthma
   attacks 45, 90
   and hygiene 32–3
   side–effects of drugs **51–2**
   treatments for 41–5, 67
atopic dermatitis 46–7
atopy 9–10
Attention Deficit Disorder (ADD) 3–4, 85–6
Ayurveda 65

babies 7–8, 13–15, 82–4
Babies' Breath 76
bathing 11, 76
beclomethasone 44
bedding 21
bifidus treatments 19
bio–resonance 59, 61, **68–70**
blood tests 39–40, 57–8, 65
breastfeeding 7, 81, 82–3
breathing techniques 73–5
Brethine 43
Bricanyl 43
bronchodilators *see* 'relievers'
budesonide 44
burdock 68
Butyeko Method 74–5

Candida albicans 6, 19, 62
carbon dioxide levels 75
chamomile 67, 76
chemical pollutants 23
Chi (energy) 65, 71, 74
childcare 87–8
coal tar ointments 46–7
colic 4, 13–14
complementary therapies 53–77
condensation 23
consultations for complementary therapies
   acupuncture 71
   eastern medicine 66
   herbalism 67
   homeopathy 63–4

naturopathy 65
nutritional therapy 61–2
conventional medicine 37–52
corticosteroid medication 46
cortisol 72–3
counselling 73
cow's milk, allergies to 7–8, 13–15, 83
crab apple 76

dairy products 5
damp 23
dance therapy 73
deafness 48
decoctions 67
desensitization 38, 48, **50**, 63–4, 86
diary keeping 16, 86
diet **7–8**, 34, 61–2, 65
doctors 37, 38, 39, 43, 55–6
double–blind trials 54
dowsing 59
drama therapy 73
dust mites 20–1

eastern medicine 65–6
echinacea 64
eczema 10–11, **46–7**, 68
electromagnetic energy 76–7
eliminations diets **40–1**, 57, 86, 95–8
ELISA (Enzyme Linked ImmunoSorbent
  Assay) 40
embarrassment, feelings of 26, 28
emergency treatment 45, 90
emotions, and allergies 25–35
energy fields 69
'energy medicine' 70
Enzyme potentiated desensitization
  (EPD) 50, 86
EpiPen 50, 90
essential oils 67, 75–6
eucalyptus oil 67
evening primrose 11
exclusion diets 16–18
eyebright 68

FACT (Food Allergy Cellular Test) 40,
  57–8
families 30–1

family medical history 9–10, 43, 63
'favourite foods' exclusion diet 16–17
fibre 62
flower remedies 76
food allergies 7–8
  self–tests for 15–18
  testing for 39–41, 57–9
food cravings 16
'food group' exclusion diet 17–18, 95–8
food intolerances **3–6**, 15–16, 49
food remedies 60, **70**
food therapies *see* nutritional therapy
frankincense 76

gardens 23–4
garlic 68
genetic links 9–10, 43, 63
geranium 76
glucuronidase 50
glutens 83
grape hyacinth 76
green rose 76
'growing out of' prognosis 38
guilt feelings 32
Gut Permeability Test 58–9 *see also*
  Leaky Gut Syndrome

hair analysis 59
hayfever 47–9, 68
headache tablets 5
healing 76–7
Health Education Authority (UK) 83
healthy diet, importance of 52
herbal medicine 66–8
hereditary predispositions 9–10
histamine 2, 50
holistic therapies *see* complementary
  therapies
home improvements 22–3
homeopathy 62–4
hormones 72
hospitalization 45, 46
household allergens 20–3
hydrocortisone 50
hydrotherapy 64
hygiene and asthma 32–3
hyperactivity 3–4, **85–6**

hypnotherapy 73

immune system 1, 2, 7, 8, 72–3
immunoglobulin E (IgE) 2, 37, 57
immunotherapy *see* desensitization
infusions 67
inhalers 26, 43, **44**
intolerances *see* food intolerances
iridology 65

kinesiology 59

La Lèche League 83
Lantana 76
laser acupuncture 72
lavender 76
Leaky Gut Syndrome 5–6, **18–19**, 58–9, 60
'leaving home' and health care 91–2
lemon balm 76
long–term drug use 44
Low Allergen Garden 23–4
Luffa 76
lunchboxes 88–9

Ma Huang 68
marigold 68
marshmallow root 67
massage 75–6
meditation 28
mega–vitamin supplements 56
Min–I–Jet 50
mould spores 23, 24, 47
music therapy 73

nasal medication 48
National Childbirth Trust (NCT) 83
naturopathy 60, **64–5**
neroli 76
nettle 68
nut allergies 1, 26–7, 31, 80–1
nutritional therapy 60, 61–2

organic produce 52, 65
over–the–counter medicine 56
oxygenesis 74

parents 29–35
peak flow meter readings 43
peanut allergies 80–1
peppermint 75
pets 22, 85
physical exercise 34, 89
pollen allergies 24, 47
pollutants 5, 6–7, 23
porridge oats 11
Prana 65
preconceptual care 80–1
prednisolone 46
prednisone 46
pregnancy 80–1
preschool children 84–8
'preventers' 44
primary school children 88–90
probifidus 19
processed foods 7
profilin 48
pseudo–allergy *see* food intolerances
psoralen 47
psychological therapies 61, **72–3**
psycho–neuro–immunology (PNI) 72
PUVA (Ultraviolet light treatment) 47

RAST (radioallergosorbent test) 39–40
raw food 65
relaxation therapies 35, 73
'relievers' 43–4, 51
remedial yoga 74

St John's Wort 68
Salbulin 43
Salbutamol 43
school, primary 88–90
self–esteem, boosting 28
self–help tests 57
Shiatsu 72
siblings 9, 30–1
side–effects of drugs 44, **51–2**
skin prick test 39
sleep 35
smoking 34–5
social occasions 27, 89
sodium benzoate 86

sodium cromoglycate (cromolyn sodium) 44, 48
solvents 23
soya products 8
sports 89
steroids 44, 45, 51, 46
stress 26, 34, 72–3, 74

t'ai chi 34
teachers 89–90
teenagers 79, **90–2**
terbutaline 43
tests for allergies 39–41, 57–9
therapists, complementary 54–6
tinctures 67
toddlers 84–8
toxins 7, 62, 64
Traditional Chinese Medicine (TCM) 65, 66, 70–1
treatments

for asthma 41–5, 67
for eczema 46–7, 68
for hayfever 47–9, 68
triggers 49–50

ultrasound acupuncture 72
urine tests 58, 65

vaccinations 10–11, 33
vacuuming 21
Ventolin 43

water consumption 62
water therapy 64
weaning 83
withdrawal symptoms 17–18

yeast organisms 6
Yin and *Yang* 62, 71
yoga 28, 34, 74

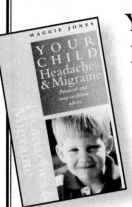

YOUR CHILD: HEADACHES AND MIGRAINE

Maggie Jones

A clear practical overview of migraine and headaches in children, from the causes to their sometimes distressing effects. Includes information on the many effective complementary approaches and self-help techniques that are available.

216 x 138 mm, 128 pages ISBN: 1 86204 397 3
£5.99 paperback US **$9.95** / CAN **$13.99**

YOUR CHILD: ASTHMA

Erika Harvey

Examines all aspects of living with a child with asthma: the treatments, the practical steps and how to cope positively.

216 x 138 mm, 136 pages
ISBN: 1 86204 207 1
£5.99 paperback US **$ 9.95** / CAN **$13.99**

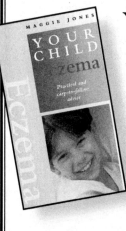

YOUR CHILD: ECZEMA

Maggie Jones

Contains the latest information on the conventional and alternative applications for eczema and highlights cases where treatment has been successful.

216 x 138 mm, 112 pages ISBN: 1 86204 209 8
£5.99 paperback US **$9.95** / CAN **$13.99**

ELEMENT

THE ELEMENT FAMILY ENCYCLOPEDIA OF HEALTH

Dr R. Sharma

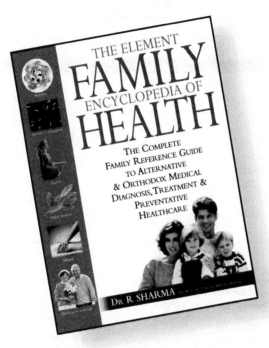

Anyone with an interest in healthcare should have this unique reference guide which covers both orthodox and complementary treatments in equal depth. This thorough and authoritative encyclopedia provides expert advice for most common medical conditions and covers all ages from conception through childhood to maturity. Contains over 200 illustrations including diagrams, charts and photographs.

255 x 189 mm,   2-colour printing with black & white illustrations,
640 pages ISBN: 1 86204 301 9
£24.99 hardback US **$34.95** / CAN **$43.99**

ELEMENT

TO ORDER

UK: Please call the credit card order line on **0870 2413065** or fax your order to **01747 851394**.
For postal orders please send a cheque or postal order made payable to Element Books, together with your name and address
and the completed order form; (photocopies accepted) to: **Element Direct, Longmead, Shaftesbury, Dorset, SP7 8PL.**
Postage & packing free. *Please quote code YR1 on all orders*

US: Please call **1 800 788 6262** or Fax: **201 896 8569**. Please have your Visa, Mastercard or American Express ready.
You will be charged at the list price plus a shipping and handling fee and any applicable sales tax.

CANADA: Orders to: **Penguin Books Canada Ltd, c/o Canbook Distribution Center,**
1220 Nicholson Road, Newmarket, Ontario L3V 7V1.
Toll-Free Customer Service
Canada-wide Tel: **1 800 399 6858** Canada-wide Fax: **1 800 363 2665** Toronto line: **905 713 3852**

TITLE	ISBN	PRICE	QUANITY	TOTAL PRICE
		TOTAL		

All UK and European trade enquiries should be directed to
Penguin Books Ltd, Bath Road, Harmondsworth, West Drayton, Middlesex. UB7 0DA. Tel: 0181 8994036
For information on Element Books and how to order them outside the UK please contact your appropriate distributor.
(Prices correct at time of going to press, all books subject to availability)

AUSTRALIA
Penguin Books Australia Ltd
487 Maroondah Highway, PO Box 257, Ringwood, Victoria
3134, Australia
Tel: (3) 9871 2400, Fax: (3) 9870 9618

NEW ZEALAND
Penguin Books New Zealand Ltd
182-190 Wairau Road, Private Bag 102902,
North Shore Mail Centre, Auckland 10, New Zealand
Tel: (9) 415 4700, Fax: (9) 415 4704
or (customer services) 444 1470

SOUTH AFRICA
Penguin Books South Africa (Pty) Ltd
Private Bag X1, Park View, 2122 Johannesburg,
South Africa
Tel: (11) 482 1520, Fax: (11) 482 6669

CENTRAL & SOUTH AMERICA
Book Business International
Rue Dr Estdras Pacheco Ferreira 200, 04507 0 060
Vila Nova Conceicao, Sao Paulo SP, Brazil
Tel: (11) 884 2198, Fax: (11) 884 2198

PHILIPPINES
Penguin Putnam Inc.
375 Hudson Street, New York, NY 10014, USA
Tel: (212) 366 2000, Fax: (212) 366 2940

INDIA, SRI LANKA & BANGLADESH
Penguin Books India Pvt Ltd
11 Community Centre, Panchsheel Park,
New Delhi 110017, India
Tel: (11) 649 4401/649 4405, Fax: (11) 649 4402

PAKISTAN
Book Com
Main Chambers, 3 Temple Road, GPO Box 518,
Lahore, Pakistan
Tel: (42) 636 7275, Fax: (42) 636 1370

JAPAN
Penguin Books Japan Ltd
Kaneko Building, 2-3-25 Koraku, Bunkyo-ku,
Tokyo 112, Japan
Tel: (3) 3815 6840, Fax: (3) 3815 6841

SOUTH EAST ASIA/FAR EAST
Penguin Books Ltd
2nd Floor, Cornwall House, Taikoo Place,
979 King's Road, Quarry Bay, Hong Kong
Tel: (852) 2 856 6448, Fax: (852) 2 579 0119

SINGAPORE
STP Distributors Pte Ltd
Books Division, Pasir Panjang Districentre, Block 1,
No. 03-01, Pasir Panjang Road, Singapore 0511
Tel: 276 7626, Fax: 276 7119

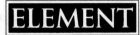